In the Land
of Forgetfulness

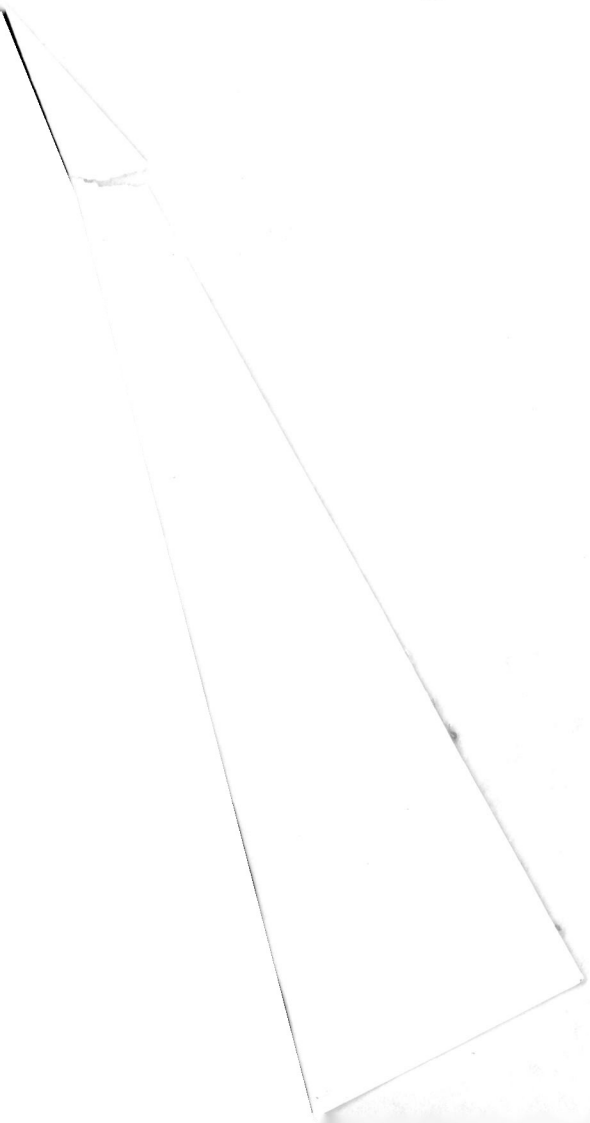

In the Land
of Forgetfulness

Meditations on Dementia Care
as Spiritual Formation

WAYNE A. EWING

Foreword by Nicole Parsons

WIPF & STOCK · Eugene, Oregon

IN THE LAND OF FORGETFULNESS
Meditations on Dementia Care as Spiritual Formation

Wipf & Stock
An Imprint of Wipf and Stock Publishers
199 W. 8th Ave., Suite 3
Eugene, OR 97401

www.wipfandstock.com

PAPERBACK ISBN: 979-8-3852-2262-9
HARDCOVER ISBN: 979-8-3852-2263-6
EBOOK ISBN: 979-8-3852-2264-3

VERSION NUMBER 07/22/24

Bible references are from The New Oxford Annotated Bible, New Revised Standard Edition Oxford University Press, 1991.

To all dementia caregivers, you who accompany the Beloved
into and through the land of forgetfulness

Are your wonders known in the darkness,
or your saving help in the land of forgetfulness?

PSALM 88:12

Contents

Foreword

I WRITE THIS FOREWORD mindful that I am only familiar with half the story this book is telling. As of this writing, I have not been on a journey of dementia caregiving. I have only been bumbling my way along the paths of spiritual formation. As a spiritual seeker and companion to other spiritual seekers, I've been gnawed by a hunger for greater intimacy with the Holy.

The thing about hunger is that it's uncomfortable and demanding. It makes us cranky to start, but left unattended, it demoralizes and immobilizes. Hunger of any kind is not a desirable state. And yet, the author of this book has a profound way of approaching such gaping ache through an unexpected door.

With compassionate precision, Wayne Ewing describes the pang that is the natural and immediate response to a diagnosis of any form of dementia in a loved one. Knowing this ache intimately, Wayne names it as dread and then makes a remarkable claim. "Dread is a spiritual state," he writes early in the book, "and [it] can be touched spiritually."

This stunning invitation to recognize a potential encounter with *mysterium tremendum et fascinans* in the journey of dementia caregiving sets the tender meditations of this book in motion. Wayne's testimony flows from his own hard-struggled experience with the slow loss of his beloved spouse, Ann. That story is told in the companion volume, *Tears in God's Bottle*.

Foreword

Here, in *In the Land of Forgetfulness*, through a series of short meditations, our author remaps the inner complexity of caregiving within another set of maps generations old. These ancient waymarks were made by centuries of contemplative people who were seeking—and finding—intimacy and union with the Numinous. In chorus with Wayne, these gentle voices extend invitations to ponder the parallels. They are wholehearted companions who have been somewhere painfully difficult, and who also have a willingness to wonder if, in such darkness, more is going on than we can know or imagine.

Wayne's spiritual curiosity leads to some profound parallels. For instance, forgetfulness, the watermark of dementia, turns out to be also a watermark of intimacy with the Holy—in the form of self-forgetfulness. A growing distance from what the world considers useful, and even a porous and non-chronological relationship with time itself—these dreaded aspects of dementia show up as "features" of increased spiritual nourishment rather than "bugs." But this is not a whitewash job. Letting go will never ever be easy in either our outer or inner lives! But there is something spacious in the suggestion that the never-sought labor of dementia caregiving could become a spiritual container, a crucible, for deeper becoming.

It is entirely conceivable that someday I will be a caregiver. This book tells me that nurturing my spiritual life right now may be one of the greatest gifts I could give my Beloved and myself in preparation for such a time. I am so grateful for this signpost.

And I trust it. I trust this message because I trust this author as a guide. I confess I don't understand all that he has to say; I have not stood where he has stood. But though I don't comprehend every word written here, I trust because I am apprehended by the idea that Wayne and his contemplative conversation partners in this book affirm: every gaping ache can be a threshold, and Love can always become its meaning.

Nicole Parsons
Westcliffe, Colorado
Summer, 2024

Historical Notes

AUGUSTINE (354–430)[1]

Of Romanized Berber origin in North Africa (present day Algeria), Augustine's mother, Monica, was a baptized Christian; his Roman gentleman father, Patricius, received baptism upon his deathbed, a common practice in that day, during Augustine's adolescence. Augustine was educated in North Africa and went on to study and teach in Milan, Italy, for some years. There he was mentored by Ambrose, accepted baptism, and upon returning to Africa in the early 390s was ordained a presbyter, similar to what we would call a "priest" today. He reluctantly became the bishop of Hippo, an ancient port city, where he remained, other than his travels, until his death. A fierce intellectual, a gifted and voluminous writer, and a respected speaker and spokesperson for the Christianity he crafted from biblical and classical philosophical sources, he shaped Christian thinking, polemics, devotion, and reflection for centuries to come. He is still much consulted and commented upon by historians of thought, philosophers, theologians, and ordinary folk drawn to his very accessible writings.

1. All dates are Common Era.

BERNARD OF CLAIRVAUX (1090–1153)

Born of Burgundian nobility, Bernard, along with scores of other young noblemen, entered monastic life in 1113 at the Benedictine chapter in Citeaux. Three years later he and a dozen other monks were sent to found a new house in the Diocese of Langres, which Bernard named Clairvaux; his name is forever inseparable from Clairvaux, where he soon became, and remained to his death, a reforming abbot. His spirituality is marked by devotion to Jesus' mother, Mary, mystical vision, and austerity of life. So powerful was he in monastic reform, however, that he was solicited as mediator and churchman into both political and theological controversies by Roman popes. Widely known throughout Europe during his lifetime, his sermons, polemical treatises, and commentaries remain in print to this day.

THE CLOUD OF UNKNOWING (LATTER HALF OF THE FOURTEENTH CENTURY)

This anonymous counsel on contemplative prayer and mysticism was written in Middle English as a guide for an inquiring student. *Cloud* promotes interior contemplation stripped of all thinking and motivated by love, in order to enter "unknowing," wherein God's love and presence are actually revealed, experienced, and quietly celebrated. The book became widely circulated and apparently has inspired contemplatives and spiritual inquirers from the near contemporary Nicolas of Cusa (see below, p. xvi) to the twenty-first-century Franciscan brother Richard Rohr, a popular and widely read spiritual counselor (see www.cac.org).

MEISTER ECKHART (1260–1328)

A German Dominican monk from late adolescence, Eckhart advanced through his order to have increasing dominance and influence as a theologian and mystic in a tumultuous time of conflict within monastic orders. Reflective of this dynamic, he was declared a heretic by a Franciscan tribunal but died before a final papal judgment was delivered. To this day his Roman Catholic "orthodoxy" is debated, while his fecund praise of, and mystical reflection within, the Holy has continually been drawn on by spiritual contemplatives and students for seven centuries.

FRANCIS DE SALES (1567–1622)

A young nobleman of Savoy, Francis was on a trajectory to become a soldier/statesman. However, through his participation in the theological controversies generated by the clash of Protestant Calvinism with Catholicism, he was drawn to consecrate himself to the Blessed Virgin Mary and to dedicate his now chaste life to God. With doctorates in both law and theology, he was ordained a priest in 1593 and assigned to Geneva, where he was eventually consecrated bishop. His ministry, preaching, and writings quietly advocated a devout life, sprinkled with openness to mystical vision. He was one of the first to write a devotional life guide for lay people; *Introduction to the Devout Life* was received well by both Catholics and Protestants and has remained in print to this day, being used as well in spiritual direction.

HILDEGARD OF BINGEN (1098–1179)

One of the most powerful and influential persons in the High Middle Ages of Western civilization, Hildegard, although a cloistered Benedictine nun and abbess, was known as a prolific author, musical composer, medical writer and practitioner, and counselor to both secular and religious leaders of her day. Her unique gifts in both early scientific inquiry and visionary, mystical theology continue to attract contemporary students, scholars, and inquirers. Canonized only in 2010, her writings, mandalas, paintings, and music have been part of the world's cultural and intellectual landscape for nine centuries.

JOHN OF THE CROSS (1542-1591)

A Spanish Roman Catholic priest, mystic, and friar of the mendicant Carmelite order, John was an instrumental voice within the Counter-Reformation. Both his poetry and his theological narratives on spiritual development are still regarded as pinnacles of Spanish Catholic mysticism. Early in his own spiritual formation he met Teresa of Avila (see below, p. xvii) and became engaged in her Carmelite reform to a more rigorous, prayerful, contemplative lifestyle. He added "of the Cross" to his name in 1568, upon his formation of a new Carmelite community in derelict church properties donated to Teresa. The reforms were contested, and John was imprisoned and tortured by resistant Carmelites; during this time and afterwards as an escapee, he produced some of his most soaring writings on the journey of the soul from darkness to light.

JULIAN OF NORWICH (1343-1416)

An "anchoress"—a woman who devoutly committed herself to living in a solitary cell (in her case, attached to the parish church of St. Julian in Norwich) in seclusion from her community—Julian lived through sieges of plague, peasant revolt, and suppression of proto-Protestant Christians in one of the most "religious" English cities of the era. When afflicted with what appeared to be a fatal illness, Julian was visited by a series of visions, or "showings," of the suffering of Jesus. She survived, as have two accounts of her visions, which are now the earliest English literary works known to be authored by a woman. Mostly unknown until the early twentieth century, Julian has emerged as a prominent and lasting contributor to the dynamics and practices of contemplative life and prayer. As Margery Kempe (see below, p. xv) witnesses, Julian was a correspondent and personal counsel to contemplatives and inquirers throughout her life.

THOMAS KEATING (1923–2018)

A Cistercian monk in the austere Trappist tradition from age twenty, Keating is one of those modern spiritual directors who contributed to the late twentieth-century renewal of interest in contemplative mysticism and prayer. It is often suggested that his seminal comment, "Silence is God's first language. Everything else is a poor translation,"[2] remains a distillation of contemplative practice and devotion in our own day.

MARGERY KEMPE (1373–1438)

Herself illiterate, Margery Kempe dictated late in her life what is regarded as the first autobiography in the English language. *The Book of Margery Kempe* relates her adult life as a woman both tormented by and assured by the Christian faith and practice of her day. The "memoir," so to speak, is also a recounting of her spiritual journey and mystic vision, one that engaged her across Europe in public testimony to, and critique of, ordinary piety. She regarded Jesus not only as the author of her salvation, but as the coauthor of her meditative reflections.

SØREN KIERKEGAARD (1813–1855)

A Danish philosopher, ethicist, and theologian, Kierkegaard was a prodigious writer, publishing, sometimes in clever pseudonyms, about fifty volumes of criticism, counsel, and sardonic reflection in a little more than a decade of authorship. Regarded as the "father of existentialism," his works also foster the sense of the individual soul in intense conflict with self, society, culture, and accepted religion. For him, faith commitments emerge both as mysterious gifts and as intellectually disciplined choices.

2. Keating, *Invitation to Love*, 90.

MECHTHILD OF MAGDEBURG (1207–1282)

Born into a noble family, the mystic poet Mechthild of Magdeburg experienced her first religious vision at age twelve, and daily apparitions appeared to her for the remainder of her life. In 1230, she became a beguine in one of a group of thousands of evangelical women of the day in that region who took vows together but lived in the world rather than a convent. She did spend the last twelve years of her life, however, in a cloistered Cistercian community. Written over fourteen years, her seven-volume book, *The Flowing Light of the Godhead*, was one of the first German mystic texts composed in vernacular Low German rather than Latin. These devotional poems, reflecting her own ecstatic divine vision and fearless critique of local clergy, may have influenced Dante's *Divine Comedy*. Her work was largely forgotten after her death until its rediscovery in the late nineteenth century. Her poetry appears in current anthologies.

NICOLAS OF CUSA (1401–1464)

Papal legate and statesman, the highly educated Nicolas found time in his travels throughout Europe to write almost thirty learned books and treatises on mathematics, astronomy, theology, and meditative discourses on spiritual formation. When named a bishop and cardinal by Pope Nicholas V, his commitment to reform led to his secular imprisonment, from which he was eventually freed by papal intervention, but from which he never fully recovered physically or pastorally. He was widely read and published and has remained as a cited authority for both secular and religious reform insights across the centuries.

RUMI (1207–1273)

Possibly the world's most widely published and read poet in literary history, Rumi was a Sunni jurist, scholar, theologian, and mystic in the Islamic Sufi tradition. He wrote mostly in Persian, although he authored some of his immense work in Turkish, Arabic, and Greek. Born in what we know as Afghanistan, he spent most of his adult and professional life in Samarkand (in modern day Uzbekistan), an influential commercial, religious, and cultural center and crossroads in the thirteenth century. His burial place in Konya (central Turkey) became a pilgrimage shrine, and his family and followers formed the Mevlevi Order, the Order of the Whirling Dervishes, whose dance is known worldwide. Rumi was of such stature that his biography is interlaced with marvelous legends.

TERESA OF AVILA (1515–1582)

The older mentor and compatriot of John of the Cross (see above, p. xiv), Teresa was instrumental in Spanish Counter-Reformation practice, devotion, and reflection. A Carmelite reformer, her writings have become classics of Christian mystical meditation. At age seven, in a passionately driven foray into secular life, she ran away with her brother to martyr herself in battle with the Moors but was retrieved from that venture by an observant uncle. Her spiritual formation was also affected by an extended illness, her miraculous recovery, and her reading one of the first Spanish translations of Augustine's *Confessions* (see above, p. xi).

Acknowledgments

"ACKNOWLEDGMENTS" SEEMS SUCH A small envelope into which I might tuck the immense gratefulness I hold in my heart for all those who have assisted me in seeing *In the Land of Forgetfulness* into publication. Imagine rather, a large ceremonial bowl chock full of slips with these eucharists:

For my household family, with whom I am blessed to live quietly on our M66 ranch, in our stunningly beautiful, isolated Colorado high mountain valley; they have seen to it that just the right music was playing while I first wrote, squirreled away in my study, then edited and reformatted in our cozy 150-year-old ranch house living room. These good people didn't have to "do" anything, they were simply present, and being supportive. And the cups of coffee at just the right time! So, thank you, Shannon Proctor, my spouse, and Charles Proctor, my ninety-eight-year-old father-in-law, for whom both Shannon and I are privileged to be caregivers.

For my extended family, some nearby in Colorado, some far afield across the country. These, too, were present with encouragement and motivating messages all along the way. The Ewing sons who also experienced their mother in the prime of her brilliant life passing into and through the land of forgetfulness: Christopher, Peter, Gregory. And my daughters-in-law, Mary, who died in hospice care while this manuscript was being proposed for publication, and Sandra Rojas, a wholistic physician who comprehends the fullness of life the ill and suffering among us actually incorporate. The grandkids and great-grandkids were always a reason to take a break and play: Lisa Ann, Isabella, Matthew, Maddie, Nathaniel, Jackson, Brooklyn Azalea, Jacob. My stepdaughter, Leah Chappabitty, who always let me know how proud she was of "Papa Wayne." My extensive in-law family, always present by nudging me on, sometimes with wild and outlandish humor: Megan and Rob, Docia and Michael, Aixe and Matthew. And then the "cuz" down the lane, Tyra, wise editor and cheerleader, whose husband Bert could be counted on to pick up any slack in meeting the physical needs of M66 while I was steeped in the book.

Then there are those who did "do" things beyond providing their welcome presence in my contemplative and writing life. The first critical readers, whose pointed suggestions I largely put into pursuant drafts: Janet Booth, Doris Dembosky, Nicole Parsons. My employers, the owners and publishers of the *Wet Mountain Tribune*, where I am honored to be a staff writer and bumbling photographer, who always gave me ample space and time to be about the work of this book: Jordan Hedberg, journalist, and his spouse, Alyssa Meier, layout and advertising specialist, both of whom are organic ranchers extraordinaire. Shannon's near lifelong friend, the LA-based Linette Padwa, who has been in the publishing industry for decades, and who shepherded me through the proposal stage of bringing the book into print.

And would that we all had a Marci Gregg in our lives; Marci came to my rescue in necessary spreadsheet preparation during the publication process.

Although they may not have realized it, the many congregants of two Colorado Episcopal faith communities, St. Luke's, Westcliffe, and St. Peter the Apostle, Pueblo have been there constantly as a nurturing, comforting, and prayerfully active resource. Peace be with you!

And for publishing itself, the Wipf and Stock staff, from our initial contact through to this finished product, have all been angels in the guise of hardworking publishers. Without editor Matthew Wimer I might have lost it at any point along the way. Kathryn Verster has been a meticulous copy editor, making the text reader-friendly; should there be any remaining errors, they are mine alone! Joe Delahanty has been very helpful in shepherding me—and my talented great-granddaughter Maddie Ewing, co-ordinator of the book's media campaign, and noted earlier in my family gratitudes—through the publicity and marketing realities of publishing. On the nuts and bolts side of business details, Emily Callihan and George Callihan have been gracious and supportive. Thank you!

Finally, and yet foremost as well, the countless people I have encountered along the way of formulating these meditations amid Alzheimer's Association, American Society of Aging, and Spirituality and Ageing conferences, those who shared the agonies and joys of their dementia caregiving, the pain and the healing of their journey with the Beloved into and through the land of forgetfulness: thank you. Were it not for your presence along the way, these reflections might never have appeared; your strength in weakness helped me immeasurably yet concretely in leading the way towards some grasp of the infinite resources available for the demanding stress of dementia caregiving.

M66
Westcliffe, Colorado
Spring, 2024

Prologue:
Where to Begin?

I FIND THAT NOT knowing exactly where to begin writing directly mimics my experience as a dementia caregiver. A profound confusion marks these opening moments. Where does one find a starting point in what appears to be an infinitely demanding journey? With what particular words might I begin these meditations on the spiritual dimensions of our experience as care partners? What could possibly be the first sentence to write while on the soulful journey of caring for someone with dementia?

Immersed in the daily, hourly chaos of uncertainty, fear, grief, and immense weariness, a dementia caregiver hardly knows where to begin the day. My only offering here is a collection of spiritual meditations. This horrid assault on the human spirit seems to demand nothing less than a spiritual response.

In a previous publication, *Tears in God's Bottle*, I shared some fumbling first steps in that direction. I wrote then from within my caregiving journey with my afflicted spouse, Ann. Over the years since her death, I have reflected further, assisted by quiet conversations with other dementia caregivers. Now I venture a few more steps.

The story that unfolds for caregivers might be compared to the launching of a newly crafted ship, down the skids from where it was built, into a channel tributary to the seven seas. Here is something already constructed, solid and massive, complete in all its systems, from the towering hull and forecastles to the tiniest screw in the galley stove. The ship is launched without a crew, however, and thus simultaneously incomplete, still awaiting the staff to run and maintain her. But then we swing the ceremonial bottle of champagne to the ship's looming side, the crew is eventually assembled, and quickly, too quickly, the ship sails on—in this instance, into vast uncharted waters.

As you might already surmise, I am constantly in quest of metaphors that might, in some slight way, capture the immensity of the spiritual passage dementia caregivers experience. I suspect that my desire to find some understandable way of expression reflects a variety of dynamics. One difficulty in writing from within the heart of experience is that perhaps not all readers will have been dementia care partners and may not grasp what I attempt to describe. Furthermore, I might need to soften somehow the harshness and jaggedness of the experience. Is there a language adequate to convey the pain and loss of dementia caregiving?

That last question is actually a motivation for even attempting to write this material. I, and the other twelve million dementia caregivers in this country, are extremely grateful for all the language available *about* caregiving. These extremely helpful and growing bodies of literature, videos, and websites provide immense commentary on the how-tos of our journey.[3] This material is produced by seriously well-intentioned professionals from many disciplines. Some of them may actually be angels in human guise—sent to let us know that we are never alone in this loneliest of personal pilgrimages.

And yet this remains language *about* caregiving. The language *of* caregiving is still in formation. Echoes, hints, and whispers of it appear in personal accounts, largely from family caregivers or persons in the "early stages" of some ghastly dementia. This is a language being birthed in the crucible of accompanying the Beloved partner, or one's own very being, into the fog of illness. The

---

3. Chief among these resources are the warmly written pages regarding caregiving on the Alzheimer's Association webpage, alz.org; sections on "Alzheimer's and Dementia" and "Help and Support" are especially significant.

words do not easily roll off the tongue, for our tongues are often numbed by the experience itself. The language we want and need to speak *of* our experience does not come readily from an ice-cold heart, an overburdened mind, or a tired body.

These are also symptoms—to borrow from a not always appropriate medical metaphor—of the great shock we tender our mind, body, and spirit when entering upon the dementia caregiving journey. You who have been and are dementia caregivers know, as I learned, that nothing in the continuum of our life experience actually prepares us for the tasks at hand. Of course there are some recognizable skills available, some remembrances of behavior that might be appropriately useful, some rekindled repertoire of activity that could prove helpful. Those of us who have parented children might also have some fall-back experience; those of us with related professional lives might bring into the here and now of our new life as caregivers a handful of relevant information. Yet for the most part, wherever we have previously been in life comes to an abrupt halt, and a newly demanding life opens before us. Somehow, the how-to manuals never seem quite congruent with the reality in front of us. Largely because that reality in front of us is our Beloved, with all this person's history and tradition, and not the dementia profile dealt with in the language *about* caregiving.

The language *about* caregiving thankfully alerts us to some of the storms ahead and the survival techniques necessary to weathering them—somewhat like a long-ago guesswork map or an imaginary navigational chart for the crew of this newly launched ship. But my experience has been that the more I was exposed to language *about* the passage ahead, the more terrified I became. For me, knowing what the journey was likely to entail, coupled with the dawning realization that I had not been trained or apprenticed for the journey, was a combination resulting in increasing, not decreasing, uncertainty and existential *angst*.

In my later life, I have been graced not only with my personal experience in dementia caregiving, but as well with the company and literature of many family caregivers from a vast array of places, circumstances and engagement.[4] I have slowly come to recognize some peculiar elements of what it is that carries us through what otherwise might be a devastating and life-taking experience. For we do come through this journey. We emerge on the other side, changed, certainly, but nonetheless somewhat intact, and still a tad familiar with our sense of self. When I pause to take inventory of what contributes to completing this strange and demanding passage and listen to the blessed company of others who ply this particular path, I am taken by what I can only describe as the growing presence of a spiritual transformation, deeply imbedded in the soul's wisdom.

I began to realize that I *had already* been exposed to a resource rich in the language of dementia caregiving. Well before I was ever aware that I would be launched onto a personal journey across this vast ocean, I had heard the pilgrims' language. I had not recognized this at the time of course, and the awareness of the resource that arose in me during the sea passage was unbidden, non-reflective, and spontaneous. I simply began to recognize the murmurs of a long-standing, ancient conversation within my immediate experience. I began to listen to the conversation, soulfully, from the inside-out. Over the years preceding my caregiving, I had tuned into the conversation from the outside in, as most of us ordinary folk do.

I was coming to learn that the language *of* dementia caregiving in fact *has* been spoken and written—but from an unsuspected, even broadly unfamiliar, source. Specifically, I became intrigued by what I was beginning to hear as the odd parallel of the caregiver's journey with the counsel of Jewish, Christian, and Islamic spiritual elders. I was astounded to discover in my listening, an uncanny similarity of our Beloved's dementia with the spiritual wisdom advocated within these Abrahamic reflections. I am, in the end, delighted to find that the otherwise dark passage we and

4. For example, John Bayley's *Elegy for Iris*, Thomas DeBaggio's *Losing My Mind*, Dasha Kiper's *Travelers to Unimaginable Lands*, and my own *Tears in God's Bottle*. Not all of us make it, however. Some years ago, a Stanford University study estimated that 41 percent of dementia caregivers die in the midst of the journey. See Living Better 50, "Startling Number."

the Beloved take together is well-lighted by the soulful presence of surprisingly accessible, powerful spiritual insight, some of which was proffered millennia ago.

I am not suggesting that becoming familiar with this strange but notable circumstance in turn becomes a way to prepare for dementia care. I continue to contend that it is unlikely that anything in the ordinariness of life would ever condition us for an extraordinary and unexpected placement into the new life of caregiving. I do suggest, however, that exposure to the elements of spiritual formation advocated by these elders help us articulate the language *of* caregiving—and that might be of some small succor for those of us who will be going there.

For that is the additional audience to caregiving concerns: those who *will be* caregivers. So many of us are temporarily abled and remain in the company of other temporarily abled people. One or the other of us—I or my Beloved—may encounter a change in that circumstance. We may enter a new place, a new land, unexpectedly and unprepared. Some of us may find this to be the Land of Forgetfulness and, like the psalmist so long ago, wonder, among other things, if there is any saving help at hand: "Are your wonders known in the darkness, or your saving help in the land of forgetfulness?" (Ps 88:12).

What follows here is meditative, not didactic, more slowly developed than quickly laid down. I have had the great good fortune to have worked for a time with a gifted stonemason and have occasionally turned my hand to garden walls with the remembrance of his mentoring and patience. A well-crafted stone structure, I learned—not only with my eyes, but also with my hands and arms and shoulders—may come together without a blueprint. However, careful attentiveness to how multiple complex shapes, with all their idiosyncratic mass, ask to be reconstituted, one with the other, can also result in a beauteous structure.

My writing, I hope, is like that. These observations of course come from my mind, but also from my heart and my spirit, from my re-membering of the muscles that ached from caregiving. I like to imagine that these quizzical, questioning, prayerful meditations are in harmony with the time and internal place of my experience as a dementia caregiver. And I also hope that these reflections might be in harmony with your own experience of how the shape, quality, and possibilities of caregiving could be affected by this particular and peculiar perspective.

As you see, I already sprinkle the words "soul," "spirit," "soulful," and "spiritual" throughout these few beginning paragraphs. I am not going to "define" these words, one by one. In the end, the dynamics and processes I attempt to point to in the common usage of these words actually define us. That is more important to me, and I hope that their usage and meanings will become translucent, a window into the puzzling experience of dementia and dementia caregiving.

I also intentionally used, and will use, "the Beloved" in reference to those we know who, before their dementia, might otherwise have born role-defined significance: partner, spouse, mother, father, grandparent, brother, sister, patient.[5] However, the persons with whom we are underway into the land of forgetfulness shed all roles and enter the blessed, sacred place of the Beloved. The Beloved is a powerful symbol and reality in the spiritual resources of the Abrahamic religions. Within these resources, the Beloved has no role definition. The Beloved is gender free, appearing as Her and Him and They. The Beloved is both source and object of the soul opened to formation, and is reverenced, not defined, is fluid, not static. In the meditations that follow, the Beloved is named in this spiritual manner. The persons who have beckoned us to accompany them on the passage into and through dementia have forsaken all roles, all definitions, and now emerge especially and gracefully as the Beloved.

So, I have chosen a beginning after all. While arbitrary, I trust it is not capricious. While there is no beginning, middle, or end in matters of the soulfully infinite, these coordinates are still important in our very temporal passage. At best handy referents, "beginning," "middle," and "end" also lose meaningful linkages to

5. I was first drawn to speaking of the Beloved in caregiving through the works of Stephen and Ondrea Levine, *Who Dies?* and *Embracing the Beloved*.

our dementia caregiving experience, and it is a good thing that the further reaches of the sacred are there to sustain us when they break away.

A final note. I am aware you are busy, engaged, even over-whelmed and stressed. Whether you are a personal or professional caregiver or friend standing by a caregiver's side, a "book" may be less than useful right now. Perhaps you could approach this material not as a "book" in the normal sense of the word, but as mentioned above, simply as the collection of meditative reflections it is. One piece a week may be enough for you. Perusing a medita-tion in the company of another caregiver may be a way to proceed. Be easy and caring with yourself, and with the meditations that follow.

Enough. Come . . .

Part One

Preparing the Spirit

THE IMMEDIATE IMMERSION INTO dementia caregiving is shockingly sudden. This is an unexpected turn in life circumstance, both for us and for our Beloved. There are quick moments of unfamiliar recognition; already the paradoxes built deeply into our journey are becoming evident. This is a crisis, a very personal crisis. It is impossible to overstate the immensity of it.

Every aspect of our lives will now be touched by a truth we had neither prepared for nor expected. Our beliefs and values, all the things that we know, are confronted by the unknown, in the company of a monstrous new reality.

Spiritually, this is an interplay of knowing and believing, one with the other. The internal spiritual processes are complex and defy simple psychologizing. Our spiritual formation may begin with these matters of stark, harsh challenge. It is a process well recognized in *The Cloud of Unknowing*, a Middle English anonymous spiritual formation treatise written in the last half of the fourteenth century. The work is conversant with a previous thousand years of commentary and reflection on approaching the Beloved.

Meditation One

Not Knowing, Not Believing

THE SYSTEMIC SHOCK OF a dementia diagnosis reverberates through both the Beloved and the loved one's partner, or adult child, or intimate friends and relatives. Even though the diagnostic trail may have been pursued for many months, it seems one is never ready for the increasing probability of diagnosis. What is this about? Diagnosis, after all, is a way of knowing something. What is it we don't want to know in this way of knowing?

It is too simple to rely on what we've learned about denial and defense mechanisms to account for an initial flight from the reality of it all. Of course we avoid bad news. We steel ourselves in all sorts of situations to repel the dreadful from our consciousness. There is nothing unique about this tendency in our human journey.

Good, solid defensiveness is almost necessary to maintain twenty-first-century life and lifestyles. I don't *want* to hear anymore bad news; my bad news quotient is filled by the time I scan or hear the first headlines of the day. Some of us have even stopped listening to, or "watching" the news. Reports of war, mayhem, violence, unnecessary death, assault, corruption and evil doings, terror, lies, and abuse fill our waking moments. So, tuning out is a measure of having mastered some sort of a minimalist survival technique. Nothing fancy, and no particular mental and spiritual gymnastic expertise is required. We simply shut out the sound and sight of the burdensome. It is too much, and we deflect it.

This is a kind of self-immunization protocol in which I imagine most, if not all, of us are well practiced. Like other forms of self-medication, we find a way to numb ourselves to what we perceive as the unpleasantness of the human journey. It is simply too painful, we say, to take on any more of the load of sorrow and mishap than what we already carry in our daily lives.

It is understandable, surely, how we and the Beloved might greet the awareness of dementia's new presence in this ordinary way. Here is my No! to the new demands of the day. Here is our indrawn protective shield against a new onslaught of information we don't *want* to incorporate into our lives.

We seem to share this kind of built-in defensive reflex with one another. What is the spiritual face of this primal dynamic in reaction to the bad news of a dementia diagnosis? "I don't *want* this!" is an exercise of will, not simply a reflex. What looks like a quick, automatic survival denial might actually be the first spiritual encounter we soulfully have with dementia. My willfulness immediately comes to the fore in connecting with this harsh reality. What seems to be a disconnect might actually be the first engaged connection we make. What seems to be a retreat from circumstance and practicality is actually my first taste of intimacy with the plight of the Beloved.

What is it I don't *want*, in choosing to take up some form of not knowing and not believing in relation to dementia? It's not really the raw news itself, is it? Somewhere, somehow, I knew it was coming anyway. The announcement might actually be a confirmation of the quietly expected, after all. We might already have entertained anticipatory scenarios of post-diagnostic life and living. Although not prepared, at some level of our experience neither are we surprised.

And yet we are shocked, thoroughly shocked. I knew the possibility was there, lurking in this march through the ever-diminishing list of possible "causes" for my Beloved's loss of cognitive ability and vibrancy. And still, the jolt is there, in the moment.

My No! is not so much denial as it is recognition. My choosing not to know and not to believe the strobe-lighted moment of this particular truth is my acceptance of dread.

I suggest that this is our ordinary way of accepting and adapting to the dreadful. This is a matter quite beyond fear and anxiety.[1] Angst and terror hardly do justice to the vast chasm into which our hearts fall in this moment of recognition. This is not a nightmare, not a dream from which I will eventually awake. This is not a symbolic moment, or an abstract entanglement with some theoretical construct of the monsters and beasts whose paths cross our lives. This is a flat-out free fall into the unknown and the incredible. It is a passage into dread. Dread is a spiritual matter.

Dread is not merely a psychological state, nor is its instantaneous introduction into our lives dealt with adequately by way of intra-psychic recourse to denial and defensiveness. Dread is a spiritual state. The willful gasp, No! comes not from my mind, but from my soul. I am not merely frightened and in some behavioral or psychological retreat. I am in dread before the unknown. My No! is an affirmation of my spiritual state.

---

1. I can't help but think of Søren Kierkegaard's *Fear and Trembling* and *The Concept of Dread*, where he moves the elements of faith psychology to spirituality.

Meditation Two

Knowing, Not Believing

ANOTHER ELEMENT OF OUR shock has to do with how many aspects of the unknown are, of course, known. There is a lot I know about the realm of dementia, even while standing in the anteroom of the unknown. I have some grasp of the turns my life will take with my Beloved.

Just as it is difficult to avoid, deliberately, the news of the day, so it is difficult in this time of increased consciousness and education *about* dementia and dementia-like disease to be ignorant of the nature of the affliction and its probable course with the Beloved. In a relatively short time, perhaps moved along by Ronald Reagan's open acknowledgment to the world of his Alzheimer's disease diagnosis in 1994,[1] vast numbers of people have come to have some idea of the demanding reaches of dementia. Dementia is not a totally unknown factor in our contemporary life.

The kind of knowing in this shared awareness can be experienced in at least two ways. One way can be understood as part of the general nature of awareness, and the other as the specific nature of awareness. Generally, awareness of something simply enters the subject, story, event, or person of our drifting attention

1. See *Newsweek's* October 1, 1995 cover story by Eleanor Clift, "The Long Goodbye"; the issue also included related articles on Alzheimer's disease.

6

into the range of the familiar. While not intimate with what we are aware of in this way—who is doing what, where, and why; what and where the main currents are in the streams of life in which we choose to participate; and so on—certainly we are not strangers to these matters either. We might be acquainted with this realm of information, or events, or remembrances, and thus know them in a passing kind of friendly neighborliness. It is more like the soft knowing of acknowledgment than it is the knowing of what we refer to as knowledge. It's something like the difference between data and significant conclusions drawn from data.

It is the other dynamic of awareness that I am concerned with here, for I think it contributes to the spiritual knowing that we couple with disbelief in confronting a dementia diagnosis. This is the awareness that is specific, pointed, concentrated on a particular matter.

Some spiritual writings speak rather clearly to being present, to paying attention, to being aware. The unknown author of the late medieval English treatise on contemplative counsel known as *The Cloud of Unknowing* actually suggests a "device" to enhance awareness. When the multitudinous frenzy of what we ordinarily "know" begins to stand in the way of our spiritual clarity, "try to look over their shoulders, as it were, looking for something else: that something else is [the Beloved], surrounded on all sides by the cloud of unknowing."[2]

Repeatedly, mystical resources like this suggest awareness— of self, of the place we occupy at the moment, of the sheer and open fact of our being in the world—as a primal step into the sacredness of life. Rumi, the much-revered thirteenth-century Sufi poet from the land we know as Afghanistan, and a near contemporary of *The Cloud of Unknowing*, says it this way:

> Notice how each particle moves.
> Notice how everyone has just arrived here from a journey.
> Notice how each wants a different food . . .
> Look at this cup that can hold the ocean.[3]

2. Walsh, *Cloud*, 181.
3. Barks, *Essential Rumi*, 7.

And there is an intimation from within Judaism that the entire rabbinic tradition can be captured in simple, focused attention.[4]

This kind of spiritual awareness, an odd way of knowing, slips into our consciousness while we walk the diagnostic path with the Beloved. But even if we do not *intend* it, specific awareness seeps into our consciousness along the way. We seem to have hidden eyes, ears, and minds that begin to see and hear and collect the details of dementia, whether we want to or not. We truly become *aware* of the dimensions of the journey ahead. It is as if we have gone on alert in some way, and a vigilance of knowing has become operative in us.

This is a spiritual experience. Somewhere we are listening to the unwanted knowledge. Somewhere we are attuned to the growing sense of what dementia can be, of what might be expected of its progression. Something in us is absorbing this knowing, even while we have our heads turned in the other direction. It is like seeing without looking; hearing without listening; becoming aware without thinking. While seemingly impossible, this is the actual dynamic of spiritual knowing. Awareness is not so much a conscious act as it is a spiritual gift. It is as if our knowing comes almost immediately into this new place in our lives in an unbidden way. I just know, we say, and the fact is, we haven't done any research, we haven't studied, we haven't been schooled. This is not intuition, however. Intuitive states are still cognitive states.

This is instead the kind of knowing awareness that comes from below, and above, and behind cognition. It is a spiritual matter, and we are gifted with a knowing that acts like a buffer between us and the harsh reality ahead of us. Soulfully, we are gathering up the knowing that eventually will be necessary to the journey.

This awareness might still be accompanied by disbelief. Again, not the disbelief of denial, but the not believing that appears with dread. For my knowing awareness is simultaneously challenging

---

4. For example, from the Mishnah tractate Avot 2:1, "Rebbi said . . . observe these three things and you will not come into the clutches of sin. Know what there is above you: an eye that sees, an ear that hears, and all your deeds are written in a book." See Taragin, "Being Aware of Awareness."

my values, my hopes, my expectations about the future. While part of me might be saying Yes! to the awareness of dementia's reality in my life, my No! still affirms my dread.

The Beloved will surely be taken hostage by the dementia. We, by the Beloved's side, are aware that our life is also captive within the new perimeters drawn by dementia. My Beloved might have no choice; I do. My No! gathers up the spiritual dread of knowing this, and simultaneously of not believing it.

Meditation Three

Not Knowing, Believing

JUST AS THERE IS a great difference between the language *about* some reality and the language *of* that reality—think of the difference between a devotional essay about prayer, and the behavior of praying—so too there is a great difference in knowing *about* something and knowing *of* it. In this shocked moment of No! confronting dementia diagnosis, whatever I know *about* dementia fades before the immensity of what I do not know *of* dementia.

Knowing awareness might still be at some safe distance, no matter how focused it is on the matters at hand. There is an aspect of not knowing, as in looking out onto the *un*known, which struggles for coherence with the accruing knowledge within me. This unknowing is all the more sharply silhouetted when accompanied by a shift in my spirit from disbelief to belief. When I choose to unleash my No! into the realm of the caregiving life suddenly thrust upon me, I am also weaving together the disparate elements of believing in the truth of what lies ahead, while blocking out the way with unknowing.

This is another indicator of the spiritual intricacy of our caregiving lives. *The Cloud of Unknowing* is exquisitely aware of this strange interweave. Speaking to one who desires to draw closer to the Beloved, the contemplative writes, "When you first begin to undertake it, all that you find is a darkness, a sort of cloud of unknowing; you cannot tell what it is. . . . This darkness and cloud is always between you and [the Beloved], no matter what you do, and it prevents you from seeing [the Beloved] clearly by the light of understanding in your reason. . . . So set yourself to rest in this darkness as long as you can, always crying out after [the Beloved]. For if you are to experience or to see [the Beloved] at all, insofar as it is possible here, it must always be in this cloud and in this darkness."[1] Perhaps you recognize yourself in these words. I certainly remember myself like this during the first weeks of our dementia journey; as this counsel suggests, I and the Beloved were in darkness.

The Cloud of Unknowing is a mirror of the mental, emotional, and spiritual jumble that I experienced. Truly, a cloud stood between me and the reality I believed I needed to embrace fully. Literally, I could not "see through" the dark cloud that had fallen down around my ordinary senses. I was wrapped in not knowing. The fog that inevitably would envelop my loved one's apparent persona was here anticipated in my own thick mists of unknowing.

And yet I share with you the profound belief that we are *to be with* the Beloved along the hazardous path ahead. *The Cloud of Unknowing* emphasizes the way belief conjoins with our unknowing: "And our soul . . . is wholly enabled to comprehend by love [the incomprehensible]. . . . You are to smite that thick cloud of unknowing with a sharp dart of longing love."[2]

"Longing love" is one way to describe the spiritual dimension of choosing to believe our new circumstances. Our belief comes to us in the form of a compassion for the Beloved. My No! is also a way of saying *not this* for my loved one and is transformed instantly into belief in the reality of it all.

My spiritual parallel with the Beloved's path incorporates a quality of protectiveness. Just as I gather a protective shield around myself with my No! so too I want to protect the Beloved from what I see lies ahead. And just as I reveal my spiritual state of dread in

1. Walsh, *Cloud*, 120–21.
2. Walsh, *Cloud*, 131.

my No! so too I reveal my spiritual state of longing love, desire, and belief in relation to the Beloved.

The spiritual nature of dementia and dementia caregiving is laid bare in the complex strata of response included in our No! My denial is an acceptance; my aversion is a knowing; my unknowing is a longing; my disbelief is an affirmation. Dread compounds all with the elements of the strange, strange circumstance of believing that which is unknowable, and knowing that which is unbelievable.

Spiritually, it is not so much a matter of finding one's way *out* of this dilemma as it is a matter of wonderment that I have found my way *into* this dilemma. After all, my belief is ordinarily something that is simply in place. My belief is rarely challenged: I simply don't allow it or expose myself much to such risk. And surely, I rest in the assurances I have surrounded myself with what I call knowledge. How odd the circumstance of dementia caregiving, that it awakens us to grapple with these two basic coordinates of personal meaning: knowing and believing.

Meditation Four

Knowing, Believing

KNOWING AND BELIEVING EVENTUALLY weave together in our caregiving. Knowledge becomes a necessary companion to our daily activities, and we find ways to enhance that knowing. We seek out literature, workshops, support groups, podcasts, and conferences. We move on from our No! to pursuits of knowledge that we might never have had occasion to think about, prior to a dementia diagnosis.

However, this affirmation of knowing needs some spiritual sustenance. If your experience is, or will be, anything like mine, this knowing can be burdensome. It is *too* much to be responsible for knowing *so* much about the dementia journey. I have often said, in very different contexts, "I wish I didn't know what I know." In *this* circumstance, our sense of being weighted down with knowing is a particularly difficult spiritual issue. That is, insofar as the knowledge we acquire is actually useful to the wide range of caregiving activities, it is a gift to us, a good gift. Yet in my hands, there are times when this gift of knowledge is unwelcome and wearying. So, spiritually, I disdain a blessing.

It is no help to me when well-intentioned friends extend me the shallow counsel to "look on the brighter side," to "accept what God wills" for me and the Beloved, to "learn the lesson" of this journey.[1] This is not spiritual counsel as understood from within spiritual writings that speak to our caregiving. If anything, it is a deflection from reality, usually for the sake of the good-hearted dispenser of these sayings, rather than for the caregiver and the Beloved. It is not to the point here, however, to psychologize or analyze the interchange of this dynamic. What is to the point is to allow the raw pain of knowing to be precisely what it is for us: a spiritual challenge. Again, the spiritual dilemma is exactly this simple acknowledgement: we inhabit an awkward space. We are stretched between naivety and despair, between not wanting to know and needing to know.

If there is any light at all in this dark place, its source is in the fire of a peculiar truth: dread is a spiritual state and can be touched spiritually. The dread I experience in my knowing No! is a familiar place for contemplatives and mystics. *The Cloud of Unknowing* even suggests that we risk bringing on our own madness, should we be nonchalant about the journey ahead of us. Using a metaphor that has chilling contemporary reality to it, the author reflects on mad-cow disease—what we know as bovine spongiform encephalopathy, BSE—as a referent for men and women who mistake their knowledge for a spiritual enthusiasm.[2]

Spiritually, the nature of knowing is powerfully demanding. It is not a simple thing, this knowing. Knowing asks us to go where we do not want to go, to use what we do not want to have, to seek what we would best fear to find. We cannot touch dread by imagining this knowing is something other than it is. In our caregiving, awareness and attention and presence bring us into an excruciatingly painful place. We touch dread, just so: No! Our knowing, while essential and necessary, alerts us to the exquisitely exposed place we now soulfully occupy. The winds of knowing blow sharply and coldly against the nakedness of our circumstances.

1. This dynamic was treated so well decades ago in Rabbi William Kushner's *When Bad Things Happen to Good People*. The fact that his observations have been so popularly received and so widely read has not mitigated, however, the offering up of this kind of "spiritual" pap.

2. Walsh, *Cloud*, 220–23.

And what about believing? Is believing the spiritual quality that brings a finely poised balance to my posture in this vulnerable place with the Beloved? I would like to think so . . . but it doesn't really work out like that. Spiritual counsel, even if using the word "simply" in relation to "believe," does not imagine a magical, fairy tale transforming instant. Rather, spiritual counsel envisions a long journey, a process perhaps unimaginably complex. *The Cloud of Unknowing*, as is common in the millennia of conversations about knowing and believing, refers to Mary, the mother of Jesus—actually, to "our Lady Saint Mary"—as an example of this virtually lifelong churning knowledge and belief focused on painful and uncertain realities. Recall that "belief" in *The Cloud of Unknowing* is also described as "longing desire," the kind of belief marked by love.

In this context, indicative of how serious the reflection on our actual spiritual state is within these resourceful traditions, the counsel speaks to the results of our awareness as humility and sorrow. If we choose to live with and through our dread, rather than ignore it or give up all hope to it, how might we go about the process?

The Cloud of Unknowing develops a peculiar, relevant response: How? Surely, just as Mary did.

> For although she could never rid herself of the deep sorrow of her Heart . . . all her lifetime she carried them with her wherever she went, as it were in a bundle bound together and stored secretly in the cavern of her heart. . . . She had a more sorrowing desire, a deeper sighing. . . . And we are not to wonder at this; for it is the nature of a true lover that the more [the lover] loves, the more [the lover] longs to love. . . . So she hung up her love and her longing desire in this cloud of unknowing, and learned to love what she could not see clearly in this life by the light of understanding in her reason.[3]

Both knowing and believing are assaulted in the shock of a diagnosis and the beginning of dementia caregiving. The strength or presence of the one is never sufficient response to the weakness

3. Walsh, *Cloud*, 153–55.

or absence of the other. Nor does the full bloom either of knowing or of believing become radiantly visible in the murky journey ahead. Their weaving together is still a tapestry of dread. In awareness of our dread, something else breaks through—and it seems to be that which lies within the Beloved's journey, not immediately in mine: love.

Spiritual writers consistently affirm that one spiritual quality alone is able to encompass, hold, and heal the spiritual reality of dread. And that is love. A mediated love in an immediate crisis.

Part Two

Dementia and the Holy

THE PARALLEL OF DEMENTIA caregiving experience with the concerns and advocacies of contemplatives and mystics is and will be woven into the fabric of these meditations. Is it simply a bizarre coincidence that the parallel can be identified? Is this often-lost caregiver's imagination grasping at the straws of remembered spiritual insights? Is this only a desperate rendering of helpless, profound pain into meaningfulness that is not actually there? A frenzied quest for solace satisfied by chimera crafted by crazed spiritual writers and counselors?

Does it matter?

Yes . . .

I find it fascinating, for a precise example, that Hildegard of Bingen's "integrative strategies" for treatment of mentally impaired people in the twelfth century is still cited in twenty-first-century scientific literature, as a mode to "move us toward a more thoroughly integrated understanding of the field[s]" of psychiatry and psychology. The "integration" of which contemporary authors speak is Hildegard's comprehension of the spiritual dimension of disorder as a necessary complement to the biological and physiological dimensions of illness.[1]

1. See Phillips and Boivin's "Medieval Holism,"; and Radden's response, "Sigewiza's Cure."

Part Two: Dementia and the Holy

I am suggesting of course that this "integration" is also a powerful dynamic within the shared experience of dementia caregiving. Let's explore now just how "integrated" these may be.

Meditation Five

The Ten Warning Signs 1–5

THERE ARE AMPLE, REPUTABLE, and readily accessible lists of Alzheimer's symptoms and behaviors, often headed by the all too ominous phrase, "warning signs."[1] I understand the intention of the phrase, yet also balk at the somewhat dramatic and hysterical tone impacted in those words. I suppose, for example, it's nice to be "warned" of impending weather, approaching wildfire, natural disaster, haphazard financial practices, and the idiosyncrasy of the visiting team's quarterback. But anticipation of disease might be more caringly described as "aids to understanding" or some such more compassionate reality, than "warnings."

Nonetheless . . .

From the array of descriptions of Alzheimer's from the outside looking in, I choose the Alzheimer's Association list, more gently titled "10 Early Signs and Symptoms of Early Alzheimer's."[2] (This list, by the way, helpfully adds an answer to "What's a typically

---

1. For example, see Lilly, "Understanding the Signs"; National Institute on Aging, "What Are the Signs?"; AARP, "10 Warning Signs"; Saling, "Understanding Alzheimer's Disease"; Mayo Clinic, "Alzheimer's Disease"; Harvard, "Warning Signs of Alzheimer's Disease." Less reputable lists are compiled by "alternative" treatment resources selling potions, supplements, etc. and often use hyperbolic words like "scary," "alert," and "shocking."

2. Alzheimer's Association, "10 Early Signs and Symptoms."

age-related change?" after each sign, thus differentiating the ordinary from the disease, and removing fear from the repertoire of response to learning about Alzheimer's.) These signs will serve us as the springboard to exploring yet more tightly the uncanny parallel of these notations with our spiritual elders' advocacy for spiritual growth and formation. So, remembering that all these signs are real and important and easily identifiable and unsettling, we move through them with our spiritual wonderment.

1. Memory loss that disrupts daily life . . . forgetting recently learned information . . . important dates or events, asking the same questions over and over, and increasingly needing to rely on memory aids (e.g., reminder notes or electronic devices) or family members for things they used to handle on their own.

In relation to the complex reflections of philosophers, theologians, psychiatrists, and psychologists exercised on memory, consciousness, and forgetfulness, spiritual contemplatives and mystics have a unique voice: they advocate forgetfulness. We have already had occasion to cite *The Cloud of Unknowing*. John of the Cross, however, is one of the clearest voices for the holiness of forgetfulness in these spiritual sources. He simply rehearses, in multiple contexts and counsels, that union with the Holy is marked by forgetting—forgetting not simply as a spiritual exercise of emptying, but actually forgetting: to eat, drink, remember tasks, what has been said, and seen. What is perceived as loss in dementia, John of the Cross repeatedly construes as gain in holiness; oblivion to the ordinary is not only the path, but the end, of sacred union. He joyously writes to one of his correspondents that in his retirement, he relishes "the delightful fruit of forgetfulness of self and of all things."[3] He has realized the culmination of his own counsel, that we be "elevated to God in forgetfulness."[4]

3. John of the Cross, *Works*, 759.
4. John of the Cross, *Works*, 339.

2. Challenges in planning or solving problems. Some
   people living with dementia may experience changes in
   their ability to develop and follow a plan or work with
   numbers.... They may have difficulty concentrating.

The spiritual counselors and confessors with whom I am familiar
construe concentration as contemplation, prayer, and accrued focus on union with the Holy. That contemplation can be broken and
go adrift is a given for them; return is by way of satisfying longing
through contrition, repentance—the essence of return, a change in
direction—and practice.

Julian of Norwich writes extensively of this experience. And
sensually so, we might note. In one of her "showings," or revela-
tions, she is given something "as small as a hazelnut" to palm, as
if it were everything that exists. Her insight? That it can "fall into
nothing" in a blink, and just as all that exists, it is present only
through grace, love, mercy. Spiritual union with the Holy, she suggests, is inhibited by undue attention to the daily matters of the ordinary world; only when union is experienced, can we "have love
or rest or true happiness." Those who are occupied "with earthly
business" cannot find rest, for "they love and seek their rest in this
thing which is so little and in which there is no rest." Julian refers
to this "blessed revelation" as one of the "nothings" with which she
has been graced "No soul has rest until it has despised as nothing
all that is created." The soul, she claims, is in turn to "become nothing for love," and thence be rewarded, at last, with rest.[5]

As for concentration, or contemplation, on these matters,
Julian notes that it is of two orders: lower—that "earthly business"
which keeps us in fear—and higher—where we are led to "spiritual
joy and true delight" in the Holy. She encourages us to maintain
knowledge of the former, for all sorts of practical and sound matters, while remaining as much as we can in the latter, where joy,
bliss, peace, and love also remain.[6]

---

5. Julian of Norwich, *Showings*, 130, 183.
6. Julian of Norwich, *Showings*, 339.

3. Difficulty completing familiar tasks. People with Alzheimer's often find it hard to complete daily tasks.

The sources referred to throughout these meditations are pretty straightforward about the valorization of daily tasks. Meister Eckhart, for example, who claims the Holy is accessible "everywhere, in the streets and in company with everyone, just as much as in church or in solitary places," nonetheless also claims that seeking or grasping the Holy "in works or people or places" is for naught. Tasks and work are of little significance in experiencing the Holy, but disposition and intention are of great significance. He illustrates this by citing those who are consumed by thirst, or possessed by love: wherever they are, or with whomever they may be, the intention to drink or to love remains within them. Just so, Eckhart points out, the Holy "does not vanish" when the intention to live in this Presence remains, above and beyond the tasks at hand.[7]

John of the Cross is even more harsh in the assessment of work in the world as it is usually understood. There is great harm in focusing on tasks, he claims, because it is a source of spiritual harm; the joy in them can be seen as an idolatry of work. To avoid the snares of "vanity, pride, vainglory, and presumption," we "must hide [our] work so that only God might see it and should . . . not want anyone to pay attention to it." Not only should our tasks be hidden from others, but even from ourselves. We are to "desire neither the complacency of esteeming [our] work as if it has value, nor the procurement of satisfaction. . . . Do not esteem with the temporal and carnal eye the spiritual work [we] do." He even construes the familiar experience of accomplishing tasks as an arena where the "self-love contained in . . . works" makes the heart cold to actual love.[8]

---

7. Colledge and McGinn, *Eckhart*, 251–53.
8. John of the Cross, *Works*, 318–20.

4. Confusion with time or place. People living with Alzheimer's can lose track of dates, seasons and the passage of time.

Sometimes they may forget where they are or how they got there. These very conditions—losing the sense of date, season, time, place—are those described by a number of the contemplatives cited as the experience they have when in the thrall and throes of unitive vision with the Holy. Even the rather heady churchman, scholar, and diplomat Nicolas of Cusa, whose musing on infinity in his *The Vision of God* can be rather mind boggling, lifts up an ejaculatory confession of being out of his mind in a chapter on "How that, unless God were Infinite, He would not be the End of Desire." In the midst of his treatise, written in 1453 at the behest of the prior and monks of the Benedictine Abbey of Tegernsee, that they might learn of him "an easy path unto mystical theology," he states, "I behold Thee, O Lord my God, in a kind of mental trance, for if sight be not sated with seeing, nor the ear with hearing, then much less is the intellect with understanding." In other words, he's lost track of where he is and what time it is, yet he is in "bliss."[9]

Even though Julian of Norwich can, and does, precisely date and place the circumstances of her visions, whilst engaged in them in great pain, pain leaves, the natural light leaves, the room and those about her leave, and in union with the Holy, she enters a timeless bliss.[10] In similar fashion, Hildegard of Bingen specifically dates the recording of her visions, naming who was archbishop, who was king, who was abbot, and yet within the visions she is lost to all else but the piercing experience itself—which is nowhere near the here and now of her very active, forceful, and creative life. In her own words:

> In the year 1141 of the incarnation of Jesus Christ, the Word of God, when I was forty-two years and seven months old, a burning light coming from heaven poured into my mind. Like a flame which does not burn but

9. Nicolas of Cusa, *Vision of God*, 76–77.
10. Julian of Norwich, *Showings*, 179–81.

rather enkindles, it inflamed my heart and my breast, just
as the sun warms something with its rays . . . I had felt
within myself the gift of secret mysteries and wondrous
visions from the time I was a little girl. . . . I revealed my
gift to no one. . . . I concealed my gift continuously in
quiet silence until God wished it to be manifest by God's
own grace. I truly saw those visions; I did not perceive
them in dreams, nor while sleeping, nor in a frenzy, nor
with the human eyes or with the external ears of a person, nor in remote places; but I received those visions
according to the will of God while I was awake and alert
with a clear mind, with the innermost eyes and ears of
a person, and in open places. . . . [A]fter I had passed
through the turning point of young womanhood, when
I had arrived at the beginning of the age of perfect forti-
tude, I again heard a heavenly voice speaking. . . . And I
spoke and wrote these things not according to the inven-
tion of my or any other person's heart, but as I saw, heard,
and perceived them in the heavens through the hidden
mysteries of God.[11]

Teresa of Avila notes, too, in *Interior Castle*, "I seem rather to
be talking nonsense. . . . But you must understand that there are
many ways of 'being' in a place"; and later, "God help me in the
mess I have gotten into!"[12] Within her vision, locked as it is in time
and place, she herself has come into a timeless and unknown place.

5. Trouble understanding visual images and spatial relationships.

In the contemplative sources cited, and to be cited, it follows then,
too, that those caught up in union with the Holy are confessedly
confused by "visual images and spatial relationships," going so far
as even to exclude what is ordinarily seen in the ordinary world.
The experienced visions are described and explicated with clarity,
yet the oddness of the interior experience itself is repeatedly noted.

11. Hozeski, *Hildegard*, ch. 9.
12. Teresa of Avila, *Interior Castle*, 31, 80.

For example, in a sermon in which he extols the wisdom of Aristotle on what makes humans human—understanding images and forms—Meister Eckhart goes on to conclude that, really, "the last end of being is the darkness or the unknownness of the hidden."[13] He contends we know not what, of what we "see" in union with the Holy. In one of his "Counsels on Discernment," Eckhart prescribes that "a man should have his inwardness well protected, and that his mind be on its guard against the images that surround him outside, keeping them out, never letting them intrude to occupy him and accompany him, never letting them find a home in him."[14]

Of her precious "showings," Julian of Norwich notes that they "cannot persist in this life," that she is led to understand that particularly disturbing visions would "pass," leaving her "with neither sign nor token whereby I could know [the revelation]," going so far as to claim that "when the vision had passed, like a wretch I denied it, and openly said I had been raving." Her only solace is that the Holy had provided the vision, and that she might continue to hold the learning therefrom "by faith."[15]

Hildegard of Bingen, under the impress of the brightness of fire and light in her visions writes that she is "not strong enough" to endure the attention of the Holy in her "weak human contemplation."[16] She is prone to ask of her visions, not simply as a rhetorical device, but as an existential bind, "What does this mean?" And there are scattered instances of "Why?" as well.[17]

These visionaries take nothing for granted in the experience of union with the Holy. The very experience, clear as it may be expressed, remains fraught, indeed, with troubled understanding.

---

13. Colledge and McGinn, *Eckhart*, 192.
14. Colledge and McGinn, *Eckhart*, 274.
15. Julian of Norwich, *Showings*, 261, 316–17.
16. Hozeski, *Hildegard*, ch. 10, Vision One, pt. 3.
17. Hozeski, *Hildegard*, ch. 11, Vision Two, pts. 5 and 27.

Meditation Six

The Ten Warning Signs 6–10

6. New problems with words in speaking or writing.
   People living with Alzheimer's . . . may repeat
   themselves. They may struggle with vocabulary, have
   trouble naming a familiar object.

CONTEMPLATIVES SEEM TO "STRUGGLE with vocabulary" with
some frequency. It is a dynamic that comes along with the desire
to express the inexpressible, to give words to the ineffable. John of
the Cross states this in a manner that is shared by other contemplatives and mystics: "In contemplation God teaches the soul very
quietly and secretly, without its knowing how, without the sound
of words." The phrasing is within his commentary on the Song of
Songs, written in 1584 for the Carmelite nuns of St. Joseph's in
Granada, in the prologue to which he had written, "And who can
express with words the experience [the Holy] imparts to thee? . . .
Certainly, no one can!"[1]

The same sense is conveyed by Teresa of Avila, who, as already
noted, severely doubts her ability to fulfill adequately the task re-
quested of her. There is no false modesty, only the fumbling way
of a contemplative, in her dedication of *Interior Castle*: "If I am

1. John of the Cross, *Works*, 626.

successful in anything that I may say, [my readers] will of course understand that it does not come from me."[2] In other words, she neither trusts her words and vocabulary, nor has any confidence she has chosen her words wisely. Meister Eckhart masterfully works through this spiritual dynamic in his "Sermon 2," where, after clearly struggling to elevate his hearers to a place where they might be open to the presence of the Holy in their lives, he has to conclude:

> I have sometimes said that there is a power in the spirit that alone is free. Sometimes I have said that it is a guard of the spirit; sometimes I have said it is a light of the spirit; sometimes I have said it is a spark. But now I say that it is neither this nor that. . . . And therefore I now give it finer names than I have ever given it before, and yet whatever fine names, whatever words we use, they are telling lies, and it is far above them.[3]

He indeed struggles with vocabulary.

7. Misplacing things and losing the ability to retrace steps. A person living with Alzheimer's disease . . . may lose things and be unable to go back over their steps to find them again.

The contemplatives cited throughout these meditations of course prefer that we have no attachment to "things" at all! Misplacing them and not being able to find them again would be of no concern. "Nothing" is not simply a vacuous reference to self-sacrifice; rather, as in the counsel of *The Cloud of Unknowing*, the nothing of spiritual striving is the "Everything" of spiritual awareness.[4]

Often, the springboard used by contemplatives for the venture into dispossession of material things, affairs, and concerns is constructed by contrasting Mary and Martha in their reception of

2. Teresa of Avila, *Interior Castle*, 25.

3. Colledge and McGinn, *Eckhart*, 180.

4. Walsh, *Cloud*, a theme repeated in chs. 17, 23, 49, 68.

their rabbi, Jesus, into their home.[5] Martha is "distracted by many things," while Mary, focusing on Jesus' presence and teaching, "has chosen the better part." So it is in *The Cloud of Unknowing*, as well as for Meister Eckhart, who identifies the "one thing necessary" that Jesus refers to in the gospel story as detachment, a virtue he elevates above love, humility, and mercifulness on the path to union with the Holy.[6] "Things" are of little or no import in these counsels regarding spiritual formation.

8. Decreased or poor judgment. Individuals may experience changes in judgment or decision-making.

The contemplatives who have been guiding us in these meditations defer judgment and discernment in all matters to the Holy, with Whom they seek union. Julian of Norwich, for example, relates the inability to attain "true judgment" to fears that lock us into untruths in general. Human judgment and discernment is, after all, quite fickle, "sometimes good and lenient, sometimes hard and painful," susceptible to "changeable sensuality, which now seems one thing, and now another."[7] Human judgment in general is not to be trusted.

John of the Cross agrees, assessing human judgment as one of those dynamics perhaps irreparably caught up in the constantly beckoning material world; indeed vanity, he suggests, harms the ability to judge and discern with any sense of appropriateness: "Reason and judgment of the spirit become very dull, as in the case of joy over temporal goods, and in some ways even duller . . . clouded by emotion." Further, the foibles of self-deceit spawn a kind of "darkened" outlook that leads us weary folk into being "extremely weak, lukewarm, and careless in knowing and practicing true judgment."[8]

5. Luke 10:38–42.
6. Colledge and McGinn, *Eckhart*, 285.
7. Julian of Norwich, *Showings*, 323, 256.
8. John of the Cross, *Works*, 306, 289.

In the spiritual formation advocated in these sources, human judgment is always suspect from the get-go, and its honing to some sort of worthiness is turned over to the Holy.

9. Withdrawal from work or social activities. A person living with Alzheimer's disease . . . may withdraw from hobbies, social activities or other engagements.

It is fairly clear that our contemplatives advocate "withdrawal" from ordinary society. It is practically seen as a necessity for spiritual formation. As already noted, Meister Eckhart finds "no other virtue better than a pure detachment from all things."[9] Within her visions Julian of Norwich is dying, even dead, to the world, even as she is led to share with us the fruits of her pain and insight to the Holy.[10] John of the Cross even contends, rather harshly, that withdrawal from the world is not in itself sufficient for spiritual formation; our own "spiritual sweet tooth" of prayer and meditation needs to be abandoned as well—"this is what loving [the Holy] means," a self-denial that includes spiritual "nakedness, poverty, selflessness . . . purity." He honors withdrawal as a spiritual "oblivion," marked by "purity and simplicity."[11] The physical image with which Nicolas of Cusa accompanies his *The Vision of God* is for the sole purpose of enticing the good monks of Tegernsee to withdraw "beyond all sight of our eyes, our reason, and understanding."[12]

Withdrawal is proffered by these contemplatives as the *sine qua non* of spiritual formation.

9. Colledge and McGinn, *Eckhart*, 285.

10. Julian of Norwich, *Showings*, 127, 179.

11. John of the Cross, *Works*, 170, 195.

12. Nicolas of Cusa, *Vision of God*, 2.

10. Changes in mood and personality. Individuals living with Alzheimer's may experience mood and personality changes. They can become confused, suspicious, depressed, fearful or anxious.

As contemplatives move deeper into spiritual formation, some seem hardly to recognize themselves. Nicolas of Cusa's exclamation that he beholds the Holy "in a kind of mental trance"[13] is of this note. Hildegard of Bingen's account of her life trajectory from childhood to the adult woman who is transported in her visions is a veritable quest for "Who am I?"[14] Both Meister Eckhart and John of the Cross lift up Paul's ecstatic—which means standing outside oneself, being displaced—claim that it is no longer he who lives, but the Holy within him,[15] as a paradigm for "complete detachment"[16] and the "intimate spiritual embrace"[17] with the Holy.

The shadow side of loss of self—fear, anxiety, depression—is reflected in Julian of Norwich's frequent reflections on despair.[18] In Teresa of Avila's interior approach to the Fifth Mansion, reflecting on loving one's neighbor, she despairs of her or her sisters ever knowing their true selves as they "must do violence" to their own wills and being.[19]

And so . . .

When my Beloved seized her head in her hands and wept aloud, for the last time, her full name and title—"I am no longer Ann Margaret Wentz Ewing, PhD"—she was inadvertently echoing, in agony, those mystified contemplatives who had lost themselves in wonder, awe, and the majesty of union with the Holy they sought.

---

13. Nicolas of Cusa, *Vision of God*, 78.

14. Hozeski, *Hildegard*, ch. 9.

15. Gal 2:20.

16. Colledge and McGinn, *Eckhart*, 288.

17. John of the Cross, *Works*, 518, 562, 671.

18. Julian of Norwich, *Showings*, 167, 322.

19. Teresa of Avila, *Interior Castle*, 111–17.

Part Three

And Where Does
the Spirit Abide . . .

SPIRITUALITY AND DEMENTIA CAREGIVING live in the same world. The possibility for our spiritual formation within the experience of dementia caregiving rests on this simple observation. We do not leave the world of caregiving to go find the world of soulful spiritual formation somewhere else. They are one and the same worlds. This awareness is another reminder of how being present and attentive is a doorway to the Spirit—and when we walk through that door, we have not at all left the actual world of our daily lives.

This observation seems to run counter to commonplace understandings of spirituality and creates difficulties in readily discussing spiritual formation in ordinary life circumstances—let alone the circumstance of dementia caregiving. Where does the spirit abide in all this worldly activity? How do I even talk *about* it, much less speak *of* it? Our spiritual elders have considered these matters for millennia. Their insights bear looking at in the light of our own immediate difficulties.

Meditation Seven

Peculiarities in Addressing
Spirit and the Spiritual

WE HAVE BEEN LIVING in a time when "spirituality" seems to be reemerging as a significant dynamic within popular concerns of mass culture.[1] That doesn't make it any easier for us, however, in speaking directly and meaningfully to spiritual matters. Many of us still have the common experience of feeling an awkward embarrassment when we bring spiritual matters into conversation. That is, of course, matched by the difficulty we may have in entering these matters in our own hearts.

Is there a special learning involved, after all? Are there particularly appropriate vocabularies and contexts—and particularly inappropriate ones? Might the realm of Spirit and spirituality actually be a very private one, one which finds no connection to others, to community?

These questions could spin out of control. They reflect not only some wondering about the special place in life of Spirit, but also a basic doubt about the connectedness of the spiritual with everyday life. Even though ample, and widely read, contemporary

---

1. Frederic and Mary Ann Brussat make an excellent commentary on this phenomenon in the introduction to their anthology *Spiritual Literacy: Reading the Sacred in Everyday Life.*

literature abounds with affirmations of this connectedness,[2] so much around us still runs screaming off in the other direction. We are exposed much more to affirmations that meaning, purposefulness, and happiness are dependent on the world of things, and stuff. There it is again: world.

World. The very word calls up images of density, mass, solidity, frenzied activity, noise, commerce. Might it be so then, that Spirit is, in fact, another quite different and separate "world," an "immaterial" world?

There is a lot of language in spiritual counsel that would seem to indicate that such is the case. Mystics do seem to tell us that there is a "leaving" involved; we are to leave the world behind.

In Hildegard von Bingen's exposition of her Vision Ten in *Scivias,* she writes of "contempt for the world" as "a Christian perfection . . . for the Son of God most clearly shows the fullness of virtue in the rejection of secular things. For He, living among humans, did not pant for earthly things; and so He admonished His imitators to strive eagerly after the heavenly."[3]

Rebbe Nachman of Bratislav relates in one of his Hasidic tales how it is that "all the pleasures in the world" cannot possibly attain to the realms of the Holy One.[4]

Meister Eckhart counsels, "Detachment . . . cleanses the soul . . . and makes her one with God. . . . If then [we are going] to be like God, so far as any creature can resemble God, it will be by detachment."[5]

Rumi muses,

> In a boat down a fast-running creek,
> it feels like trees on the bank
> are rushing by. What seems

2. Again, the work of the Brussats, but also the writings of Thomas Moore, Marianne Williamson, Ken Wilber, Thich Nhat Hanh, the Dalai Lama, Edward Hayes, et al.

3. Hozeski, *Hildegard*, Vision Ten, pts. 13, 21, 26.

4. Band, *Nachman*, 221.

5. Colledge and McGinn, *Eckhart*, 144.

to be changing around us
is rather the speed of our craft
leaving this world.[6]

Yet the wonderful truth is that each one of the mystics quoted here were quite immersed in the world of human, material affairs. Hildegard was gloriously engaged in worldly affairs—all the way from supervising construction to musical composition to pharmaceutical research. Rebbe Nachman was enmeshed in all the tensions of political and competitive, charismatic problems of religious life and leadership in Poland. Meister Eckhart was, in effect, the Dominican dean of studies at the University of Cologne and may have died while walking five hundred miles to Avignon to clear his name of heresy. Rumi, even in moving from his life as sheikh and religious scholar to dervish poet and singer, clung to the matters of ordinary human life and living.

If these good folk never "left the world," whatever are they talking about? It is especially important to have a sense of what their referents are if we begin to regard their way of looking at life as inherent in, and contributive to, the dynamics of dementia caregiving. Symbol and metaphor are at work here. There *is* a journey involved. Yet, obviously, neither these mystics nor we caregivers are drifting off some so-called "material plane" to an invisible "spiritual plane." That's metaphysics, not spirituality. There is, however, a particular journeying or movement deep within the world of ordinary experience to which these spiritual writers point. It is not so much that the world in which we live must yield in some way to Spirit, as it is that our movement within the world is everywhere imbued with Spirit:

> . . . the Holy Ghost
> o'er the bent world broods
> with warm breast and ah!
> bright wings.[7]

6. Barks, *Essential Rumi*, 194.
7. Hopkins, "God's Grandeur."

Even though Gerard Manly Hopkins's words continue to loan themselves to that sense of two separate realms, we may also hear them as references to the inclusion of one sensitivity within another, both grounded right here and now. Not separation, but union; not differentiation, but sameness. Not dualistic, but unitive. It just takes a bit of moving around, attentively, in the world. The journey is *here*, not *from* here.

Certainly our Beloved is journeying, yet not going anywhere. The fixedness of the dementia journey is something we don't often speak of, yet is quite central to our caregiving experience. The world seems to become smaller and smaller and smaller for the Beloved. The great world of experience and memory and history and tradition—all this broad range of reference—seems to shrink, finally, to this particular room or chair or window to this particularly repeated story or phrase or sound. Even though we want to say the Beloved has "left" us, or "gone into her own world," or "retreated from the world," nothing could be more painfully obvious than that the Beloved and I are right *here*, now.

I suggest that's what our mystic friends are talking about. We don't really go anywhere. We are not counseled to leave one world for another. There is *here*, and although we might yearn for *there*—whether it be heaven, or the presence of God, paradise, or restored pre-dementia health and well-being—there is no passage from one *to* the other. The passage, the journey, is taking place in the one place that matters: the world we have, the world we have been given, the world that knows no other way to identify itself than as the body of the sacred.

Perhaps that is what is really peculiar about referencing the soulfully spiritual in our everyday experience. All those other concerns expressed in my initial, tumbling questions are on the surface. Within the depths is the dawning realization that to speak in ordinary ways, attentively, to our ordinary worlds—including the world of dementia caregiving—is to speak of Spirit. That, I suggest, is the only peculiarity of expression involved—and it's not terribly peculiar! We are not engaged with matters of unique differentness removed *from* here. Rather, we are simply engaged with the uniqueness of *here*. This place is already filled, before me, with Spirit—awaiting to be born anew.

Meditation Eight

The Very Air We Breathe

WHEN MY BELOVED AND I began our journey in dementia care, and as I became more aware of the spiritual richness impregnating our days, one hour at a time, several of my friends challenged the way in which I was framing our time together. The gist of their critique was basically some form of an old philosophical canard, "If everything is spiritual, then nothing is spiritual." These were friendly conversations, and intended to be supportive, helpful even, as my friends apparently wanted me to be more "real," or grounded in "practical matters." A way into these conversations from a different tack occurred to me rather suddenly one day, when a friend said, "Wayne, it's like grabbing air!"

Ah, precisely . . .

We grab air every living moment, awake or asleep, consciously or simply autonomically, and we have organs for it: lungs. The wisdom impacted in ancient languages had long ago made an intimate connection of body and spirit in the physicality of breathing. Way before it dawned on me that linguistic resources were available to describe and explore the realm of dementia caregiving, Sanskrit, Hebrew, and Greek each had found a tongue to speak meaningfully of the visitation of Spirit in the very air we breathe. In each of these languages, words that designate breath also are pointers to a more vast, immaterial world of Spirit. And it can be no accident that it takes a particular push of breath and breathing to vocalize the word in each of these languages.

The word חורה (*ruach*) appears almost four hundred times in Hebrew scripture, referring repeatedly to both God's breathing Spirit or human breathing. The wind that sweeps over the waters in the creation mythology of Gen 1:2 is *ruach*; the wind that divides the waters for the Hebrew slaves escaping Egypt is *ruach*; the breath that enlivens lifeless bodies (Ezek 37:9–10) is *ruach*; the breath gifted to the living (Isa 42:5) is *ruach*; even Job's repulsive bad breath (Job 19:17) is *ruach*; the creative power of life itself (Ps 33:6) is *ruach*.

Note, too, that a speaker/reader needs to lung-drive the speaking of *ruach*, in order to close the word on its hard guttural. It is necessary to focus on our breath to speak aloud of spiritual dimensions and presence.

The Greek equivalent of *ruach* is πνεῦμα (*pneuma*), and also serves to translate its Hebrew counterpart. The two linguistically share an identical range of meaning across breath, breathing, and spirit. In one striking instance—the Gospel of John 3:8—the dual reference to an external wind and the abiding presence of God is expressed in a single sentence: "The wind [*pneuma*] blows where it will, and you hear the sound of it, but you do not know from where it comes; so it is with everyone born of the Spirit [Πνεύματος, *pneumatos*]." In the Gospel of Matthew's account of Jesus' death, he cries out and yields up his *pneuma*; either or both breath and spirit satisfy the writer's intent. In the poem known as the Magnificat, it is Mary's *pneuma* that rejoices. The possibility of human relationship with the transcendent sacred is described as *pneuma* in several Greek New Testament passages, especially in Rom 8:16, where Paul writes, "The Spirit testifies to our spirit that we are children of God." In the almost four hundred instances of the use of *pneuma* in the Greek New Testament, the ease of understanding the intertwining of our human breath with a sacred, spiritual realm or presence is repeatedly demonstrated.

And as is the case with Hebrew, so too with Greek. It takes breath to express spirit, *pneuma*. While in English the *p* is silent in "pneumatic" and "pneumonia," this is not the case in Greek pronunciation. The *p* is hard, and the speaker must push the word *pneuma* forward, must breathe the expression of spirit into life.

प्राण (*prana*) is an equally complex reference to both breathing and spiritual presence, not only in Sanskrit, but in Prakrit, Marathi, Pali, and Hindi as well, with profound significance for those who practice Buddhism, or observe Hindu or Jainist spiritual disciplines. In American life, many students engaged in any one of the variety of yoga practices available here will recognize *prana*. Some scholars and spiritual leaders regard *prana* as non-translatable, yet the function of the word, like *ruach* and *pneuma*, is similar: a reference to spiritual life force that is also expressible in breath and breathing. And again, the soft vocalization of *prana* is a breath outward after an inhalation.

There is no coincidence involved here. No matter how we choose to understand the formation of languages geographically, anatomically, intellectually, neuro-developmentally, it seems clear that from ancient times, across disparate and distant Semitic, Greek, and Indo-Aryan cultures, our elders deeply appreciated the interwoven dynamics of breathing and the spiritual dimensions of life. These shared meanings allow me, allow us, to similarly deeply appreciate that "grabbing air" is a function of ordinary life that is simultaneously lifted into spiritual realities.

Meditation Nine

The Organ of the Spirit

WHAT IS TO THE spirit, then, as our lungs are to breathing? If there is to be more than just a curious factoid attached to the ancient linguistic duality of spirit and breath, we need to be able to answer that question. The dynamic pointed to in the ancient words is beyond metaphor, beyond poetic device, beyond a teaching moment—although each of these is a function of awesomely intertwined meanings.

Early on in my caregiving journey with my Beloved, my spouse Ann, I received an unexpected but most welcome phone call from our friend Charlie Baldwin. Charlie was then Brown University Chaplain, a former mentor and supervisor of my seminary internship, some thirty years previously. He was responding lovingly to a letter I had written lifting up our dementia caregiving journey. He dearly loved Ann, was enthralled by her ferocious wit and straightforward approach to life, and cherished her candid assessment of the matters that would occupy, say, a university chaplain. He wept. I wept with him. Through his tears, he said, "Wayne, Alzheimer's is not a disease of the belly or the bone, like cancer, where we have something to fight and something to fight it with . . . it's a disease of the soul."

Part Three: And Where Does the Spirit Abide . . .

In the moment, and in the flow of our intimate and heartfelt conversation, his comment had made sense . . . until later, reflecting on and absorbing our exchange, it didn't. There was something wrong in Charlie's word picture. I wrestled with what I was sensing and feeling, finally coming to realize that Alzheimer's is not "a disease of the soul," but a soulful disease.

Alzheimer's is a brain disease, a devastating neurological storm, and as of this writing, its etiology still escapes us. We can describe it, but not know it; as indicated in earlier meditations here, we can explain it, but not understand anything about the onslaught experienced by the person whose brain is so assaulted. We can even take a scan of the diseased brain, and see only the tangles, not the adversity experienced by the person whose brain is thus revealed and imaged.

I do understand, though, how Charlie, like I, schooled and captive to Western theologies and philosophies, so readily could, in the cadence of his grief, see Ann's plight as a disease of the soul. After all, even the likes of a Augustine had sited the soul as the seat of memory.[1] His imagery has stuck. Both his *Confessions* and *On the Trinity* have been influential texts on reflection on these matters for millennia. Augustine developed a complex commentary on memory, moving it from an access to God to an analogue for the person of God. No matter how we understand Augustine's philosophical theology in Western intellectual history, no matter how much someone might delight in the Neoplatonic flow of his reflections, the simple conclusions follow: when memory goes, the soul goes; when memory goes, God leaves.

We are neither theologians nor philosophers nor historians of ideas and their impact on cultures. We are *here*, holding the hand of the Beloved in the daily daze of lost minutes and hours, with the simply impossible role of being compass and guide through the fog layered over the Beloved's landscape. And to entertain the suggestion, while looking into the clouded yet focused eye of the Beloved, that he or she has been bereft of soul, abandoned by God, is unconscionable. It not only cannot be so, in fact it is not so . . .

1. Teske, "Augustine's Philosophy"; Coleman, "Augustine's De Trinitate."

How? Those moments when the window to our Beloved's inner life is open, and the breeze of the past, long-gone or immediate, flows into our beleaguered moment, are soulful moments . . . times when the full reach of the disease is experienced existentially, and mourned for its possession of the Beloved's grasp of time and circumstance. Whatever else soul might mean to us, our Beloved's soul, as we functionally embrace it in life's daily doings, is a personal realm beyond the reach and containment of the afflictions of our Beloved's body. It shall not and is not breached by the disease. The diagnosis is confined to bodily matters, to the material of cells and neurons. Where we have previously engaged the Beloved in our love, our mutual love, so we remain . . . it is a soulful matter.

As our Beloveds' caregivers, we are not committing ourselves to a concept, or to a theology, or to a philosophy, or to some profound understanding of the Western brain/mind dilemma, or to dictionary-like definitions of soul. No. We are committing ourselves to comfort and accompany our Beloved into and through an illness. Our presence within the moments of the journey is part of our own wholeness, just as the wholeness of our Beloved is affected by the disease that has brought us here. It is an ordinary, though gut-wrenching, adult realization to come to terms with the awareness that we are larger than the sum of our parts—and we don't even know all the parts. Of course a heart beat is a heart beat, but not just a heart beat. Looking into the eyes of the Beloved is a retinal event, but not just a retinal event. In late 2022, Hal Blumenfeld, the Mark Loughridge and Michelle Williams Professor of Neurology at Yale, along with several colleagues published research findings in the journal *Nature Communications*: "Human visual consciousness involves large-scale cortical and subcortical networks independent of task report and eye movement activity." Blumenfeld's professional focus has been human consciousness, which he describes as "what makes us human . . . and it's still a mystery of modern science." He has found that some neural mechanisms involved in vision shed light on this mystery; he summarizes these current findings by noting, "The eyes are truly the window to our souls."[2] Yes.

Our bodies and our physical activities are so much more than the certain and fixed measurements we place upon them. The truth of us is always a surprise, yet does not come from nowhere. We have been gifted to speak of this realm as soul, as soulful—a dimension immeasurable, yet experienced. A mystery, perhaps as great as human consciousness itself—yet illuminated by the extraordinary loving in engaged caregiving.

As our lungs are to breathing, so our soul is to spirit, the musculature of our spirituality. Our Beloveds and we are entwined in a soulful journey.

2. Hathaway, "Eyes Offer a Window."

Meditation Ten

Exercising Spiritual Muscle

JUST AS THERE ARE a myriad of resources for those who want to develop their physical bodies—strength, balance, heart health, stamina—so too there are for those who would like to grow and nurture their spirituality. Dementia caregivers often find that our physical disciplines for health and well-being are reduced to walking. If that is exercised with the Beloved, it becomes an increasingly slower, shorter walk. And sheer physical exhaustion begins to inhibit setting aside any daily time for spiritual exercises, had that been a part of our pre-caregiving lives, or a newly desired respite.

There is a much bandied-about quotation attributed to Francis de Sales: "Half an hour's meditation each day is essential, except when you are busy. Then a full hour is needed."[1] Cute, yes. But

---

1. In *Introduction to the Devout Life*, Francis does write, "Give an hour every day to meditation before dinner; if you can, let it be early in the morning, when your mind will be less encumbered, and fresh after the night's rest. Do not spend more than an hour thus, unless specially advised to do so" (pt. 2, ch. 1). Otherwise, he seems pretty realistic about the folks for whom he writes, advising, for example, that if you've put off your prayers and meditations to later in the day, don't try after a meal: "You will perhaps be drowsy." And of course, he does promote "resolution to do better the next day." Even more realistically, he also writes, "If all these exercises were to be performed every day they would undoubtedly fill up all our time, but it is only necessary to use them according to time and place as they are wanted" (pt. 5, ch. 17).

how much of an impact does the thrust of that decorative state-ment have on the user? What sort of counsel is that, really, in the hustle-bustle twenty-first century? Who, from the comfort of an already quiet place, dares to suggest replacing our busyness with meditation?

I'm sure we kind of "get it." Slow down, be still, look inward, pray more, not less, and so on. I have not been able to trace the immediate context of the Francis quotation; it is sometimes in-troduced simply as, "Francis de Sales once said . . ." or some such reference. In the overall context of what we think we know about his life and writings, however, the quote is simply a pointer to his advocacy for Catholic Counter-Reformation devotion. His most well-known work, *Introduction to a Devout Life*, is precisely that—encouragement for those outside of ecclesiastical orders to pursue holiness within the world.

And there is that contemplation/action kicker once again—the apparently competing worlds of within and without. Again, should we caregivers allow ourselves, even in our weariness, to reframe these allusions, not only might we make better sense of Francis's counsel, we might actually be able to follow it. Let us imagine, for example, that these verbal indicators are not to com-peting realms, not even to complementary realms, but simply an acknowledgement of what life in the world feels like. "Busy" ap-plies to every moment of ordinary life, even when we're sleeping. Conscious or unconscious, our bodies are literally "at work," even when "at rest."

If the body is perpetually active, so is the soul, the organ of our spirit, and source of our spiritual nurture. We never not breathe—until, of course, we don't. One of the ordinary spiritual practices recommended by our spiritual elders and mentors is simply called "breath prayer." Put that in your search engine and you'll be "busy" for days. Yes, "simple" as it sounds, there are regimens and rou-tines, recommended remembrances of helpful words and word-ings, exploratory and instructional YouTube videos, and whole courses in developing this practice. It's a good and fine spiritual practice, but like all spiritual practices, there is complexity within the devotional observance, all of it indeed helpful, even enlightening. Breath prayer, as inviting as it is as a go-to exercise, seems still beyond the reach of the relentless demands of dementia caregiving and caregivers. Where is there time, apart from this service to and with the Beloved, for developing anything spiritually new at all?

OK, Francis, we're coming back to you. You are on to something after all. It just takes a little reckoning with how time stretches, shrinks, disappears, bursts back, recedes, flows, speeds up. Time is only a constant in its measurement, not in our experience of it (like it's taking me "forever" to formulate this meditation!). If we disallow a measure of time—half hour, hour—to frame our exercise, and allow Francis to be playful with us—as this comment surely is—there appears to be a very real possibility that our busyness in caregiving is already a spiritual exercise. For dementia caregivers, Francis's counsel could not be considered at all as a directive to "more" time for spiritual exercise. But as a parable, a swoop into our consciousness, his counsel is filled with caring love for us.

How so? One of my theological mentors from long ago and far away, Joseph Sittler, used to speak with us seminarians of the "impossible possibility" of that good news with which we were struggling to be engaged. The ordinary circumstances of life are such that the language and dynamic of faith are often beyond the reach of ordinary perception. What emerges as extraordinary then is the realization—momentary as it may be—that both language and dynamic click into meaningful and purposeful presence: what was perceived as impossible, now in gifted moments drops into the darkness of pain and suffering as an aurora of shimmering light.

Hope takes a shape, love simply happens, and where an abyss of helplessness once occupied all of our vision, the sudden, solid ground of a soulful journey presents itself for the sure footing of our next step. Perhaps the blessed impossibility that enters our experience is simply acknowledging that we had very little to do with it: we were just gracefully there.

So then with Francis's counsel. There is nothing unusual about his observation about ordinary daily life cluttered with busy, busy, busy activity, some of it to almost robotic ends. What is unusual, though, is the proffered impossibility of easing into more inner, prayerful time while immersed in this clutter. For dementia caregivers, however, the possible alights with stunning clarity: this attentiveness to the Beloved, this weariness of intense engagement, this bewildering hour with the Beloved is already our prayer, our soulful inwardness of an increase in prayerfulness. We have become, already, the impossible possibility. The exercise of our spiritual muscle has long been underway.

Part Four

The Ecosystem of the Soulful in Caregiving

EACH OF THE DISCRETE moments of dementia caregiving are, beyond the immediate perception of the caregiver, woven into an immense tapestry of compassion, unintended tenderness, and the wobbly presence of love. We stand too close to the tapestry, in the urgency of our caring, to see the pattern.

Leaving aside the metaphor of tapestry for a more current dynamic with which twenty-first-century people have become increasingly familiar, it may be helpful to think of the totality of our caregiving environment as an ecosystem. We are engaged at any given moment with a part of that larger whole but are usually disengaged from any sense of that larger whole.

These forming meditations are suggestions that the linchpin in the ecosystem—what holds the often indiscernible, complex whole together—is the gift of spiritual formation. And the gifted, of course, is the caregiver, in the daily, hourly presence of the Beloved.

Within the ecosystem of caregiving there is no aspect of life left untouched by the journey. Every life experience of the caregiver is gathered up in the caregiver's unexpected odyssey with the loved one.

Meditation Eleven

Physical and Cognitive Attentiveness

WE DEMENTIA CAREGIVERS ARE most likely to first note the heightened sense of physical constraints on our lives, and how we stretch the ordinariness of our own cognitive abilities in adapting to these constraints.

For example, the coffee table that has long been part of the household décor, perhaps even a treasured family possession, now becomes a hazard. The table's sharp corners are now a menace to a stumbling stroll through the living room. And so it is with all furniture: is the bed height appropriate to midnight awakenings; is the comfortable chair actually comfortable any longer, or has it become a challenge to the Beloved's sitting and rising; are the very dimensions of the conveniently familiar household now emerging as a landscape more treacherous than pleasant? When the Beloved pauses at the edge of the rug, stymied, it is probable that the once recognizable patterns have jumbled into a puzzling, endangering maze of holes, bumps, and boulders. The chime of the old clock, the ring of the iPhone, may all become sounds that no longer calmly alert the Beloved to familiar matters, but rather frighten, confuse, or further disorient.

So too for household items long taken for granted, their presence hardly noticed, so ordinary have they been. But now . . . where are the kitchen knives? Are they within the caregiver's reach, but out of the Beloved's? And items never before thought of as slippery or difficult, now in the Beloved's hands become sources of frustration, anger, embarrassment: the toothpaste, the jelly jar, the coffee mug. Cherished jewelry? Necklaces, wristwatches, rings, earrings, brooches, pendants all present as risky objects.

In some respects, our customary adult environment is being rebuilt backwards, and our remembrances of child-proofing rooms kicks in as a reborn competency in protecting the Beloved. The way we know things is changing; our cognitive abilities both shrink and expand—shrink by narrowing the focus of attentiveness, expand by the wisdoms of adapting the physical environment to the diminishing capabilities of the Beloved. We don't build a new house or apartment, we don't refurbish rooms one by one, we don't replace furniture en masse or empty the Beloved's drawers of long owned personal items. Rather, our minds grow as the Beloved's contracts; we reshape our thinking to accommodate the Beloved's needs.

Accompanying this version of physicality, though, is yet another aspect of the physical world and the objects within it: the holder of spacetime itself. For dementia caregivers the spacetime continuum is not a mathematical model, but the very dimension of caregiving hours. The physicality of time appears in such small matters as medical or therapy appointments, medication schedules, the remembered viewing of a non-streamed TV show that still brings delight. Numerous physical matters need to be tended to in order to be on time. This physicality appears in larger matters too. How is a wedding anniversary celebrated when only one of the partners—the caregiver—is cognizant of the significance and pathos of the date. The measure is so much more fraught with meaning than a mere number would indicate. Intimate history, embedded habits, old stories have been impacted into this simple date. The same for birthdays, or traditions of reunions, and treasured holidays. There comes a time now for the physical adjustment to, and of, time itself.

Perhaps for the first time in our lives, we become acutely aware of the universal fabric that wraps us all in the daily activities of living and being in this mysterious world we have attempted to demystify by measuring and labeling. We have learned something new about very ancient human matters.

As noted earlier in reflections on *The Cloud of Unknowing*, our cognition is expanding to incorporate this newness in ways that enhance smoothing the otherwise oh-so-rough journey. We become expert in following research and treatment protocols, in diet and nutrition, in arranging and planning comforting events, or conversely, in being diplomats of cancellations, postponements, and disappointments. This kind of cognitive attentiveness is a sort of mindfulness that moves us beyond the self. It is as if we now have two souls, two minds in our caregiver's body. We have picked up the compass and clock our Beloved has lost; we bring into our own consciousness, tired as we may be, the soulful remembrances our Beloved has given over to the enshrouding mist.

We could of course choose to view our minds as becoming increasingly taxed, overwhelmed, on the brink of breaking under the weight of dual responsibility and accountability—to self, to the Beloved, to family, to close-in friends, to medical and therapeutic teams. Yet we simultaneously have an opportunity to cherish all this new learning and knowing as the increase of spirited engagement, a freshening of cognition, a recreating of the boundaries of our faulty knowledge. Who would have known that we caregivers were to become, for most of us later in life, youngsters once again in the schoolrooms of caring . . .

We didn't ask for this. We were chosen. In accepting, we have entered upon a journey into strange territory, yes . . . but accepting this circumstance also gifts us with new minds, new consciousness, newly constructed space and time. Not the new heavens and a new earth of imagined theophanies and apocalyptic recreations; rather, the newness of spirit touched by awareness born far beyond us and brought forward as light into our darkness.

Or, as *The Cloud of Unknowing* puts it, commenting on the unexpected "sweetness" that arrives in the midst of strenuous endeavors, "what produces this pleasure is the devout stirring of love, that dwells in pure spirit."[1]

1. Walsh, *Cloud*, 72.

Meditation Twelve

Emotional Panoramas

WE DEMENTIA CAREGIVERS EXPERIENCE tumbling, sometimes disorienting, sweeps of emotion. Feelings sometimes erupt, volcanically; sometimes arise slowly, the moon-driven tide of the heart. Sometimes overwhelming, most times unsettling, yet on occasion a rare, welcome oasis in the desert our mind roams.

Perhaps we were somewhat prepared for the emotional sojourn to which we were introduced in our caregiving, either by previous experience or by exposure to counsels of expectations in regards to caregiving. No matter though. For the most part our emotions arrive raw, unprocessed, with some driven life of their own over which, in these circumstances, we have little or no control. Although it is ordinary enough to refer to "the full gamut of emotion" in contemplating dementia caregiving, there are affective experiences which defy ordinary naming. What is it that hammers in my chest, shortens and shallows my very breathing, moistens my eyes, closes down hearing anything other than the quickening pulse in every part of my body when my Beloved looks intently at me, and says "I don't know who you are"? Does the intensity of that complex feeling have a name? The experience seems beyond sadness, fear, anger: a wordless sense of erasure.

There is some benefit, though, in pausing to consider the discrete emotions which we can identify, to sort out the complexity by naming what we can name. The order of sadness, fear, anger is just as good a place to start as any. Sadness like unto no other we have ever felt perhaps. I found it very difficult to share with family and friends the profound reaches of sorrow that washed over me. I sometimes tried out familiar Scripture passages, thinking they might provide a window into my felt sadness: "O that my head were a spring of water, and my eyes a fountain of tears, so that I might weep day and night" (Jer 9:1). Well, that wasn't very effective. Nor could I very well ask my friends to read the book of Lamentations and think of me. What came close were the more familiar words penned by the ancient Greek playwright, Aeschylus; in his *Agamemnon*, the chorus laments in these words, called up by Robert Kennedy upon the tragedy of Martin Luther King Jr.'s assassination:

> Even in our sleep, pain which cannot forget
> falls drop by drop upon the heart
> until, in our own despair, against our will,
> comes wisdom through the awful grace of God.[1]

Yes, close . . . but that's all. Ordinary measures of our sorrow simply do not fit the experience of caregivers as their loved ones disappear, while remaining. Our experience cannot be grasped by reference to weight, dimension, immersion, absorption of interior space.

What then? The feeling simply remains unnamed in our trampled garden. Even though our tears may express our sadness, there is an incomplete whole, still, in this outward, visible sign of the inward, visceral terror of our sorrow. So, here it is: fear. No ordinary fear, as this thief we call dementia is a new presence in our daily lives. The wily thief is murderous, we know the thief's intent. What the thief steals is not the stuff of life, it is the love of our life. This is not the fear of fear and trembling; this is raw fear, unfiltered by any previous experience, the fear that the next unpredictable moment of our journey holds within it

---

1. Aeschylus, *Agamemnon*, line 180.

55

assaults on our consciousness *so* unimaginable as to be the dark beast of our undoing.

The anger not only knocks on the door of our sorrow and terror, it tears the door down and roars into the room of our contained experience. And while coursing through these moments of rage, a certain righteousness enfolds our being here, now, with our feeling. Helpless and futile perhaps, but righteous nonetheless. We have earned our way to anger, and no number of consolations to "calm down" are going to touch our emotion.

Where is there consolation? These are emotions so overpowering that the caregiver can become hopelessly lost: where to be with sadness, where to turn in fear, where to strike out in anger? One small, very small, consolation is an aspect of the environment of righteousness within which we feel what we feel: there is no negative or positive emotion, no right or wrong emotion, no reactive emotion to be judged by self or others. How we behave with our feelings, yes, that's up for judgment, remorse, repentance. But our emotional life in the circumstance of dementia caregiving is simply and profoundly where we find ourselves. To be affectless would be a matter of such deep denial as to undermine effective caregiving.

Is that sufficient, then, simply looking into the roiling sea of our emotions, and accepting it is what it is? Of course not. Acknowledging though that our emotions are painfully engaged in our caregiving does confirm that every facet of our life is affected by our caregiving. Here is a circumstance in our living where our emotions, as in other pre-caregiving times, are not an escape. They are entrance, full and frontally to our soulful journey itself. Sorrow, fear, anger, unnamed and precious feelings, tactile in our breath and pulse and body temp, envelop us in healthy ways—that is, as a soulful part of our wholeness. In our feelings, complex and unsettling as they may be, we are invested with the spiritual means to move with our Beloved from this despairing moment to the next, where the awful grace of the Holy appears.

Meditation Thirteen

Social and Moral Values

No MATTER WHAT WE say to and in the world, our values are evident in our behaviors. Values are enacted; if our values are not visible, whatever "value" we might be espousing could be anything—wishful thinking, a possibility for good, a theory, an opinion—but it is not a value.

Dementia caregivers experience our values, formed and incarnated in however our messy, beautiful lives may have been before caregiving, existentially confronted on a daily basis. For example, what we may previously have been engaged in that embodied our social justice values might simply go by the wayside. When attention is given to the care of the Beloved, there is little space for anything else, either physically or emotionally. Action in the world for the causes we had been promoting and advocating now becomes a matter of the past. Our social values are, at the very least, on hold. Though actually, most of us are not leaning forward into an imagined time of restoration; pre-caregiving dynamics are simply replaced by this new structure of our time and space. The future is defined not by a return to the past, but by constant immersion in the relentless present.

This is a loss in our lives. What we cared for has been replaced by the singular reality of the Beloved and the Beloved's needs.

Perhaps there is some translation or transformation of these values into our caregiving activities. After all, our compassion, even our anger, is not created from nothing; our behaviors now are still informed by what has lodged with us, with what remains from our pre-caregiving formation and experience. Nonetheless, the change in the daily routines we now invest with our energy is a change that frequently reminds us of the now forsaken environments in which we exercised social justice values.

But perhaps the even more severe assault on our values occurs when we are reminded not of social values, but of our moral and ethical values. The most pervasive moments of this dynamic are impacted in making decisions for the Beloved, whose capacity for doing so is diminished. We have to face it: it is one thing to be our Beloved's compass in space and time; it is another to be the Beloved's moral compass. It may be a matter of fiscal accountability and responsibility, especially if clear wishes had not been expressed before the Beloved slipped away. I was fortunate to have accompanied my Beloved on her dementia journey in a very small, rural community. There had been some end-of-life matters not tended to, and when it was necessary to execute some power of attorney affairs well beyond Ann's cognitive capabilities, only the compassion of a local bank officer fully aware of our plight made it possible to acquire her signatures; in a larger, anonymous, urban setting this simply may not have been possible. But yes, we caregivers find ourselves in situations where we are not only acting on behalf of our Beloved, but as our Beloved. Our moral and ethical perimeters expand into areas never travelled before.

In some specific caregiving trials, there are very private moments when our ethical values are front and center. Common to us is wrestling with truth. We are not, as the saying goes, one of those described as "a born liar." If anything, we are born truth-tellers. So, when Ann asks me in the midst of a midnight ramble through our home, "Where's my father?," I do not tell her the truth. I lie, deliberately, consciously, boldly. It is not for me to tell her that Carl is long dead these many years, and that we scattered his ashes on South Mountain. The truth would most likely create confusion or sorrow or needless argument. So I lie. "Oh, you know Carl; he thinks we don't know he still smokes, so he stepped outside for a cigarette, the devil! Would you like a cup of tea?" And the moment passes.

Those who kindly counsel us caregivers have taught us to acknowledge this lying as "creative diversion." Yet the repeated experience of such redirections tugs sharply at our ethical values; we are not liars . . . until now. On the other end of this particular ethical spectrum are those instances where we express truth in its brutality. Perhaps a family member is in harmful denial regarding the state and needs of the Beloved. Harsh as it may be, we use the hammer of truth to nail the actualities of the Beloved's dementia journey to the wall of our family member's consciousness. Or again in the intimacy of another lost day with the Beloved, the matter of truth in its starkness is expressed. As remembered earlier in these meditations, the night Ann sat bolt upright from a restless sleep, tightly clenched her head, and loudly moaned, "I am no longer Ann Margaret Wentz Ewing, PhD!," I did not argue or mollycoddle. . . . I agreed, and we wept together. When Ann would tell me that she had been "cheated, cheated, cheated" by this disease, I did not counter with some pap. She had been. We wept yet again.

One of the late medieval spiritual wanderers, the soul-tortured and controversial Margery Kempe, dictated her life and visions to scribes who thus created the first English language autobiography, *The Book of Margery Kempe.* Generally acknowledged as a mystic, others describe her simply as an oddball and uncommitted lunatic. No matter what one thinks of her, though, she at least had the clarity of imagination to render dreamlike conversations with the risen Christ into a fairly engaging read. The singular quality of most of these conversations is the topsy-turvy nature of assessing behaviors with ordinary moral and ethical assessment. What is valued as morally appropriate in the rote thoughtlessness of daily life simply is not so within the profound wrestling Margery engages in while weeping, sometimes boisterously, her way through one public suffering after another. In her "ghostly" senses, she "hears" Jesus say to her "No, no, daughter, for that thing that I love the best, they do not love: shame, insult, scorn and rebuke from the people, and therefore they shall not have this grace. For daughter, I tell you, whoever dreads the shames of the world, may not perfectly love God. And, daughter, much wickedness is hidden under the guise of holiness. Daughter, if you saw the wickedness that is wrought in the world as I do, you should have great wonder that I not take utter vengeance on them. But, daughter, I spare for your love. You weep so every day for mercy, so I must grant it to you, and the people will not believe the goodness that I work for them in you. . . . Daughter, this pleases Me, for the more shame and more scorn that you receive for the love of Me, the more joy you shall have."[1]

I happen to think of her and her literary legacy here simply because this personal revelation is an instance of the way ordinary morality and social and ethical values are construed differently, even sacredly, in immersion in pain as life flows on. And our lives, yes, flow on . . . as does our pain in love for the Beloved.

1. Kempe, *Kempe*, 208, 238.

Meditation Fourteen

Infinite Needs, Finite Resources

So, as every facet of our lives is touched and changed in our caregiving journey with the Beloved, days are filled, and filled again, with the presence we bring forward, hour by hour. So much so, that the terrain ahead seems unbounded. There is no pause or delete button we might push; we are not composed of three eight-hour shifts but have become 24/7 people. The sense that begins to pervade our experience, our being and doing in the world, is that we are confronted with infinite demands—there is an unending quality to the here and now, and the next minute, the next hour, the next day. We are being asked to meet progressively expanding, infinitely accruing caregiving necessities.

In the course of a single day, we may be asked to sacrifice every aspect of our known self to the unknown of our Beloved's need. From a love that is lost we create anew a love that will be continually exhausted and then reborn in the instant the Beloved stumbles, cries out, or retreats into silence. The round is not merely demanding; the round is repetitive and, oddly enough, unpredictable.

I remember that early in my caregiving, a person who served on the staff of the local Alzheimer's Association handed me a packet of information she was sure would be helpful. She was caring,

deeply sincere, and committed to her responsibility to be resourceful and supportive for family caregivers. She was all of that, and
to this day I am grateful for her presence at that time. And yet . . .

When I opened the packet, the sheet of paper on top astounded me. I laughed aloud, and then cried. The list before me read
"101 Things To Do with an Alzheimer's Patient." (I just checked; at
least one version of this sort of list is still available online.[1]) What
I was overcome with was an overwhelming sense of my real need:
to come through the next fifteen minutes with my Beloved with
some sense of comfort and safety for both of us. I knew that even
within that quarter hour, such a brief span of time, some wrinkle
in the flow, some sudden rapid in the stream, would appear, and I
would be unprepared. I am glad, I suppose, that the list existed and
still exists; in the rare quiet times we caregivers have to ourselves,
running through such a list may indeed be helpful. From "Listening to music" to "Ask about the person's first car," hopeful, creative
activities tick along from the world of normalcy and ordinariness.

The premiere agency designed to assist dementia caregivers
noted here just a few sentences ago, the Alzheimer's Association,
has tempered that simple listing approach over the almost fifty
years of its existence. For example, their website, www.alz.org, is
now chock full of counsel, under the overarching concern to "live
well." Daily activities, self-care, stress reduction, additional caregiver health matters, and so on, are clearly and precisely presented.
I realize in my here and now, I have time, space, energy to look into
these suggestions and guides and learn from them still. I remain
a bit anxious though about the here and now of active caregivers.

No matter how well-intentioned these Alzheimer's Association entries are, the stark reality remains that these are time-limit-
ed, finite resources for the infinitely enlarging matters at hand. Our
exhaustion is preceded by our awareness of never really coming to
the end of a day; the night remains, and then sunrise. It's as if the
biblical prophets and psalmists cry, "How long, O Lord, how long"
takes on our own version of some unanswerable plea; our lament

2. Amazingsusan, "101 Activities."

might even be soundless, voiceless, a plaintive interior ache: How long, how long?

In terms of spiritual nurture, however, we just may be confronted with one of those impossible possibilities. Perhaps we might turn this nagging sensation around, reverse the bind we feel, and flip this overbearing environment of caregiving upside down. The pain expressed in the biblical plaint "how long?" is almost always responded to with mercy and love. Perhaps our overture may be similarly addressed . . .

Part Five

From Exhaustion to Restoration

It is difficult for us caregivers, immersed as we are in the ever-changing demeanor and activities of the Beloved, to render our own changes in anything other than somewhat negative terms. The losses we see in our Beloved we translate into our own losses. The future we had imagined has become a daily engagement with needfulness and physically demanding care. We absorb the diminishment of the Beloved as our own.

The weight of hours and days bends our emotional and spiritual life into the shapes of despair and fear. Afflictive feelings seem to dominate. Softer moments that might call up joy or gratefulness quickly fade away; the light they bring don't bear up for long in the darkness. What does linger longer are those dynamics of sheer physical and spiritual exhaustion: overwhelming sorrow, stressful anxiety, anticipation only of repeated and increased diminution.

That this downward spiral in body, mind, and spirit could be reversed, could take an upward wind, could open possibilities afresh rather than close down the familiar and comforting, rarely presents itself to dementia caregivers. But yet it may be so . . .

Meditation Fifteen

Naming the Journey

I REMEMBER STILL THE moments in which I was made aware of how differently my experience as my Beloved's caregiver might be framed. It began with a phone conversation with my mother early in the months of our then despairing journey. My parents, living on a graduated senior care campus in south central Pennsylvania, and I in a rather isolated high mountain valley in Colorado, spoke with each other every Saturday. These were pre-cell phone days, when the nuances of voice were detectable—unlike our now familiar texting or FaceTime, where emojis or facial expressions assist our "hearing" the other. I am an only child, and I knew the variations in my mother's vocalizing quite well. She did most of the talking, my father coming on the line only late in the call to exchange pleasantries and assurances.

On this particular spring Saturday, I heard a somber note in my mother's inquiries about Ann and myself, about how the week had been for us. So I asked, "Mom, what's up? I can hear something's troubling you." "Son," she replied, "yesterday I was diagnosed with an inoperable, malignant brain tumor, I have three months to live." I remember a sensation much like being underwater for too long without a breathing apparatus; perhaps I even stopped breathing. I know there were further words, yet my primary recall is of the sound of silence that follows thunder in a darkening summer storm, before the lightning flash. I do know I assured her, Ann still being capable of travel, that we would be there, soon. And so we did monthly flights from Denver to Philadelphia, rented cars . . .

On the third, and final, trip—my mother died three months from the day of her diagnosis, shortly after her eightieth birthday—I accompanied her in the chauffeured senior facility van to the nearby clinic where she was receiving radiation treatment. The hope was that the treatments were relieving her of some pressure and pain; I never knew if they were or not, but it was something to do in resistance to this assault. This was a day for which the word "gray" had been created: a heavy late spring fog shrouded everything, including my mood. The red barns were gray, the budding apple orchards were gray, my mother, slumped in her wheelchair, was gray.

After wheeling her into the waiting room, and gathering up some sense of settling in for the appointment, I kneeled down beside her. My tongue was fat, my mouth was brittle dry, my breathing was shallow, my heart a block of black ice in my chest. I forced a happy face, and said, "Hey, Mom, how're ya doin'!"

My mother sat bolt upright in her wheelchair, quickly smoothed her skirt, pulled her sweater more fittingly around her, finger brushed her wispy hair into place; she knew her son had just asked her the stupidest, most insensitive question possible. She said, her eyes snapping, her voice loud enough for everyone in the waiting room to hear, loud enough for the front office staff behind the sliding glass counter pane to hear, and, should they be fortunate, loud enough for the attendant technicians, nurses, and physicians in the depths of the clinic to hear, "Son, I am not afraid!" She had spoken directly to what she had seen in me: raw, unmitigated fear. And she added, "I am only going where God has gone before."

See, here's the thing. Read carefully: my mother did not believe that. I'm her only child; I knew her in that moment with the clarity of one who has been loved to life. My mother did not believe that. No. She was so far beyond this puny thing we call "belief" that the searing impact of her words broke open my spirit to actually hear what she had just told me. She didn't believe because she had no need to believe. She knew. She was simply making a report from the fire of her immediate experience, from the sure and certain path of her painful dying. This, Son, is how it is, and a love mightier than my fear is the bright light of this dark day.

In that moment I learned how to be a caregiver. Not as in doing the "how-tos" of caregiving. Rather, I learned how to *be* a caregiver: how being in the world could be attitudinally consecrated to a path of empowering love. This journey was not contained at all in the phrase I had been using to describe it, a "dementia caregiving" journey. Ann after all was much more than her diagnosis, and the path ahead of us, the path on which we had already begun our faltering steps, was much more than a matter of coping with and managing a diagnosis. Our journey deserved a more comprehensive, comprehending name. And so I began to construe our journey as my mother had so ferociously, without guile, named it, a journey marked by a great and abounding love, a love simply given over to a bitter and suffering world, and to a pained and broken body. Perhaps that should be written, Love . . .

Further, what my mother taught me in that bright, cascading, revelatory moment was that I, like she, was not participating in an infinitely demanding circumstance at all. This journey, like all human journeys, was finite. It has a beginning, a middle, an end. The beginning was startling, unexpected, life-changing for both of us. The beginning could be recognized, and even shared with family and friends. We had begun and were now in the agonizing middle way, some directions known, some unknown. The middle was simultaneously charted in general, and unexplored in what its particular detail might be. But here we were. And the journey would have an end. Death.

Facing the reality anew, gifted by the frank assessment my mother had delivered only days from her death, I began to frame our journey as it was: a finite experience . . . for which there, indeed, may be infinite resources.

Meditation Sixteen

Reversals and Wonder

MOST OF US ARE quite aware of the power attitude has over our ordinary, daily behaviors. Our actions are tainted, sometimes subtly to be sure, and sometimes not so subtly, by the outlook we bring to the day, or hour, or moment. Our moods are affected as well, and sometimes are simply the harmony our consciousness plays with internally voiced attitudes.

I was caught up short one wearying day when I was shampooing my Beloved's hair. She was being very patient with my initial clumsiness and simply and quietly yielding to my awkward ministrations. What came to me was the realization that this was the first time I had ever done this . . .

That realization stood in stark contrast to how I had been experiencing myself in these early months of my journey with my Beloved in her dementia, our journey unfolding one day at a time with increasing debilitation and needfulness. I had been accruing quite a list of "last" things and had been dwelling on them with some consistency. I suppose I was thinking that this somehow honored our past together, our history, our traditions. Maybe so, maybe so . . . Yet what I was really doing with myself in this near daily exercise was digging a deeper and darker hole of remembrance. It was depressing. I was depressed, perhaps even clinically.

My attitude towards my caregiving was being shaped by this listing of lasts: the last time we shared a laugh over something genuinely silly and funny, a terrible joke or word pun; the last time we pranced together with our toddler granddaughter, both of us squealing like the happy kid she was in our shared play; the last time we chose a gift together for one of our adult boys, scratching our heads over what he might actually need or want; the last time we attended a large, celebrative gathering. (The latter happened to be our twenty-fifth high school class reunion, in a lovely lodge in Pennsylvania's Pocono Mountains. Ann was one of the hits of the occasion, proudly wearing her name tag upside down; when a classmate from long ago and far away would point that out, Ann, with an infectious laugh, would say, "Of course! That's so I can look to see who I am!" The poignancy of her humor was not lost on any of us.)

The list wore on: the last time we worshiped together in our historic Episcopal parish—it was an Ash Wednesday, and though my tears are differently salted now so many years later, I still weep in remembrance; the last time we collaborated on a family event, or a luncheon menu for friends invited to our mountain cabin; the last time we compared notes on a book we were reading together; the last time we shopped for our granddaughter; the last time we made love . . .

Yet in that gifted moment when I allowed myself to acknowledge I was doing something with my Beloved for the first time, another dynamic of dementia caregiving shifted beneath my feet. The earth did not move, as we say, but the way I stood upon the earth did move. Already I had come through some firsts without consecrating the moment as I might have. I realized I could instantly put that list together in a flash of recall: the first time I had actually dressed my Beloved, even choosing the outfit, in the new process trimming her wardrobe to what seemed best for our days; the first time I held a fork to her lips, because it had suddenly become unwieldy for her; the first time I had responded to any number of new questions—"Who is that?"—in the person's presence; "When do we expect Christopher [our oldest son, who lived not too distantly from us]?," when he was in the next room; when my Beloved had wearied of reading, but still yearned for a book, the first time I read aloud to her, a biography of Eleanor Roosevelt; the first time I coated and gloved and scarfed and hatted her, as the season turned and the day chilled for our daily walk . . .

That list, too, wore on. And as it did, my attitude towards many aspects of our daily life together changed. This list was not depressing; this listing became delightful, even fanciful—who would have thought I would have so many new things to learn, to experience, to catalogue, to remember, to pass on to our sons. My attitude shifted from one affected by my looking backwards and mourning to one affected by anticipation and wonder. It's just like cocking one's head a bit and seeing, even from a very slightly adjusted perspective, a fresh detail in a favorite painting—try something as familiar as da Vinci's *Mona Lisa*, lifting one's eyes from her eyes to the contrasting background landscapes, where yet an entirely different mystery comes off the canvas to greet us.

This transformation of attitude, mood, perspective, outlook on the day refreshed me. I feel I didn't "do" anything, or force something into consciousness. This conversion, a turn-around, was a soulful, spiritual matter.

I had experienced a reversal unforeseen, or thought through, or willfully coerced intellectually. This happened, unbidden, while my hands were wet and soapy, and I was task-oriented, wondering if I was "doing" this shampoo thing correctly. My being was affected, not my doing. Reshaping my attitude from looking always to the "lasts," to the simple looking into the "firsts" opened a spiritual avenue on our journey I had not seen in the making. Now that I did, there was yet another dimension of caregiving along this trying way, and a freshness was made available in the midst of my weariness.

Rumi writes,

> When I am with you, we stay up all night.
> When you're not here, I can't go to sleep.
> Praise God for these two insomnias!

And the difference between them.[1]

Yes. The difference between them, and here, the wonder of bending the very nature of caregiving time by allowing a shift in attitude to displace dispiritedness with blessing.

---

1. Barks, *Essential Rumi*, 106.

Meditation Seventeen

Prayerfulness

As TIME AND BEING took on newly different sensations and shapes for me in our caregiving journey, yet another variation on prayer and prayerfulness soulfully appeared. I had already accepted that in the absence of "taking time" for prayer and meditation, the presence to the Beloved was in fact the daily prayer—and it was a long one. But simply melding this together, as in the Benedictine *laborare est orare*, doesn't capture the spiritual fullness of our caregiving. Even the wisest of commentators seem to present this dynamic as an ideological mindset of some sort.[1] Perhaps it is, but in our caregiving experience, it cannot be only that.

Some years after Ann's death, I participated weekly in a men's contemplative prayer group, where I began to learn to name the experience we have in dementia caregiving. Central to the practice of the group were the writings of the late Father Thomas Keating, a Cistercian monk who during the years of our group's existence

1. A touching example of practice in this classic Benedictine principle is found in the calm resources presented within thecloisteredheart.org. Appropriately, from my perspective, making a monastery within, no matter who we are or where we are or how we walk in life, is a noble spiritual venture and is one of those disciplines referred to earlier as an exercise of spiritual muscle. With our meditative focus on dementia caregiving, however, we are in a spiritual environment where we seem to learn more from what happens to us, than we do by applying spiritual principles to what is happening around us.

was living in a hermitage at St. Benedict's Monastery in Snowmass, Colorado. In reading some of his long-developed reflections, and in turn, meditating on them, I realized that, most likely unknown to him, he was describing a general practice that was quite ordinary, almost a default, for dementia caregivers.

Always careful not to place contemplation and action in a false binary dichotomy, Keating frequently sketched out the various entries into, and experience within, contemplative prayer. As I came to understand him, Keating was demonstrating in his life and works that contemplative prayer is more than a calling, more than a practice, more than a willful consciousness—although each and all of those dynamics are involved. In effect he is suggesting that the fullest expression of our humanness is participation in the Holy, even though we might not name it that. He of course, did so name it, but never seemed to demand that anyone else had to do so.

"By opening yourself to God," he writes, ". . . you are accepting all reality, beginning with God and with that part of your own reality of which you may not be generally aware, namely, the spirituality of your being."[2] In passage after passage, Keating reveals a graciousness of simple acceptance for what he perceives as reality. Hey, this is the way it is, ya know? Just embrace it, walk into it, get the feel of it, be your actual, given self. He calls that the "authentic" self, but that may be a tired word for us.

We might describe our entrance into this part of our experience in another way. We're not Cistercian monks. Our form of expression may be something like this: by opening ourselves to all the vulnerabilities and demands of dementia caregiving, we are accepting a reality, beginning with the Beloved, in whose presence a yet larger reality unfolds—the Holy.

It seems to me that is the way we caregivers might eventually come to behave: when resistance and denial prove futile, we step at last into the fully given of the here and now, and we take on something real about ourselves and the world, that had not earlier in our lives been so. We are caregivers. For Keating that movement is a spiritual matter, a soulful grasp of the intentionality that

2. Keating, *Open Mind*, 43.

parallels the wonders and mysteries of all of life. In simpler words, we don't have to go anywhere special to be on a spiritual journey. Saying Yes! to our circumstances is sufficient, as painful as that may be, as sorrowful as that may be, as demanding as that may be. And in directly spiritual terms, it is both simply and profoundly a consecration of the moment—renewed every moment. Consent.

Is that not how we are in the presence of the Beloved? Consenting to the directions of meeting needfulness? This, too, in our caregiving circumstances, is how prayer—our presence with the Beloved—is transformed into prayerfulness. Being prayerful is not confined to the *act* of prayer but expands into the *being* of prayer, the rhythm of consent lifted into harmony with the fullness, as Keating was wont to say, "of the whole of creation." We are already engaged in a journey that is much larger than ourselves and our Beloved, much larger than—and certainly not confined to—this devastating dementia diagnosis. Perhaps we did not expect that the vision of that immensity would include the territory of the Holy, the mystery embedded in all of life. But here we are . . .

Keating also contends that the fullest form of prayerfulness is silence, "God's first language."[3] Moving into a personal, intimate, interior space where words, thoughts, feelings are immersed in the quieted soulfulness of intense focus in the moment at hand is an ordinary experience for dementia caregivers in our extraordinary journey. The pre-epiphany silences that move through and within the busyness of our caregiving are just that—for the epiphany does occur, the showing, the lighting of the next moment as an unexpected glory. From supposedly nowhere, the Beloved says, "Thank you, I don't know who you are, but I know I am safe with you . . ."

Reflect a moment. Is it not so that our view of reality has changed over our time of caregiving? Is it not so that our awareness has been restructured to accommodate this newer view? Is it not so that our increased sensitivity to what lies unspoken in every moment of our silent journey allows for the sudden lightning strike of union with some wholeness beyond our grasp? But not beyond our experience . . .

1. Keating, *Open Mind*, 57.

Prayerfulness

The space we occupy with the Beloved is a sacred space, and our being within this sacred space is marked by prayerfulness. Our unworded, silent prayer is lifted simply by our being here, now, with the Beloved.

Meditation Eighteen

Beginnings of Gifts[1]

WE DEMENTIA CAREGIVERS ARE rarely in a space where we think
of ourselves as receiving. After all, the operative word in how the
world describes us, labels us, is "giver." And give we do.

In the turning, though, to an attitudinal reframing of our
journey with the Beloved, there emerges the possibility of experiencing all our "giving" as simply the platform for receiving—the
gifts of our giving just may come back to us in the form of consecrated graces. Again, unexpected, spiritual gifts may arrive unbidden, unannounced, just suddenly *there* as a Presence within our
focused presence to the Beloved.

Ann and I did our utmost to walk around our mountain
fastness at least daily, if not twice a day. Weather permitting, we
traversed, at whatever the Beloved's pace was at the particular
time, a roughly one-mile path that circled through ponderosa forest and open meadow. From the outset of this near-daily routine,
Ann would pause along the way to caress a pine branch, to smell
a wildflower, to admire the glint of a quartz vein in a boulder, to
listen for wildlife, to relish the sighting of deer, to be enraptured by
burbling birdsong.

---

1. The occasions for this meditation are also detailed in Ewing, *Tears*, ch.
10, "Giving Thanks."

Just as the walks were repetitive in their own way—the same path, the same direction, the same views, the same aspen trees—Ann became repetitive in a patterned ritual, over and over again praising the environment around us. At first, I simply thought, *Yes, sure, this is to be expected, it's part of the disease in her brain.* I would quietly stand by her side, mute, while she continuously reiterated her liturgies: Such a lovely flower! Feel the softness of these pine needles! The shadow on the far mountain, so sharp! And to the deer, always: Please stay, you are so beautiful!

I realized then, and I myself repeat now, that in these moments I had a choice, one that dementia caregivers are confronted with several times a day. We can choose to become impatient, to give in to the weariness of listening to constant, monotonous speech, to hasten along the movement of this time. I could choose to say, "C'mon, Ann, let's keep walking, we want to get back before sunset . . ." Or, "You saw that flower just a minute ago, so alright already, let's move on . . ."

But I didn't.

I chose to remain silent, or sometimes ventured a simple affirmation of the Beloved's accolades and mini-celebrations. And in my silence, the poignancy of Ann's frozen recasting of sameness—moment after moment after moment, again and again and again—began to take on a dimension I had not foreseen: a dimension of spiritual nurturing, spiritual formation. For what was really going on here was much more than an Alzheimer's patient trapped in time and space and limited language. What was unfolding minute by minute was a profound witness to a reality so many of us, caregiver or not, do not care to dwell on with much reflection: this is *all* we have, this single moment. This is all that I have, this tiny capsule of time, into which is impacted all of what has been, and from which all else to be will unfold.

There is a plentitude of psychological and therapeutic commentary available on the healthy benefit of staying focused on "the here and now."[2] What I'm familiar with is helpful—good stuff. Yet

2. Clayton, "Beware of the Spiritual Abyss"; Rabb, "What Is Spiritual Bypassing?"; Welwood, *Psychology of Awakening.*

the dimensions we enter with the Beloved in our dementia care-giving journey seem to be places where most psychologists and therapists don't really go with us: spiritual space, a sacred place, say that arena where a spiritual director might nudge her or his conversant. This is a place visited with frequency on our journey with the Beloved. The pause and repetition, wherein the echo of the Beloved's voice reverberates in the soul: this moment is the gift.

The Cloud of Unknowing belabors "this nothing," "this no-where" of immediate spiritual awareness, encouraging those who choose to remain in the moment to realize the preciousness of the gift—this you have and none else, and it is filled for you, and as it is not dependent on you, it comes to you by the agilities of grace, total gift.[3] This is not a fleeting moment, but a fulfilled moment. Allowing the language of a soul on fire living within the heat of the repeated reminder that this is not only *where* we are with the Beloved, but *who* we are, eternity has left the clock and taken up all the space on this path through the ponderosa.

I could not have "arrived" at this juncture on my own; I could not have "learned" the conversion of impatience to insight by myself. I had a teacher, a spiritual guide, who happened to be an innocently ill, broken human being—herself now existing in worlds made anew every moment, herself participating in an ever-evolving landscape of perpetual novelty. I saw Ann's courage in these repetitive actions: seizing with thanksgiving what she herself had not expected—a tiny cinquefoil, a pine cone, a ray of sunshine, a fresh sound in the quiet airs of the forest. When *The Cloud of Unknowing*, in its own sing-songy repetitive way, points to "na-ked awareness," I have no better analogue for understanding than these experiences of the Beloved gathering up the fullness of time in simple praise—over and over and over again. How courageous of spirit for Ann not to have collapsed under the onslaught of con-stant stimulation, and to choose praise over confusion or pretend knowledge or fear . . . and to say: See? See? See?

I am blessed to have received the gift of hearing when I had only been listening, the gift of seeing when I had only been looking.

3. Walsh, *Cloud*, chs. 67–70.

And so may it be, with wherever the beginnings of gifts appear on our journey. They are there, awaiting . . .

Part Six

Spiritual Formations

WE LIVE IN AN era of haste to move on to what's next. The ambience of this rush to the coming moment is fed and nurtured by massive entertainment systems, as well as the constancy of social media. Hundreds of thousands of Americans, perhaps millions, go to bed with perpetual news-feed companions in hand so as not to miss anything. So many of us seem to have an aching desire not to be left out of the perpetual information loop about famous political or athletic or media people's doings, even in so-called "real time."

Real time? Familiar to gamers since the 1980s as a particular group play strategy, "real-time" has wandered into popular speech as a reference to the right-here-right-now-you-can-be-there quality that marks our haste to the next "new" thing. The qualities of quiet aging seem to be left to the ruminations of holistic gerontologists, vintners, and distillers. Far removed in feel and sense from the here and now we considered in the last meditations, this haste for the next is frenetic, with no desire to pause, remain, calmly absorb. Instant replay and slo-mo, whether on the stadium jumbotron or the home flat screen, is a poignant parody of contemplative pause, and remaining silently in the moment. Our lived environment is not inviting to the processes of spirituality and exploring spiritual growth.

However, rather than lament and encourage nostalgia for some imagined past, we have the opportunity simply to lift up this environment as our contemporary version of the "world." No matter how human haste has seemed to quicken exponentially in our time, it has always been so. Our particular challenges to spiritual processes that are much slower than the pace of life around us are simply that—our particular challenges in the environment of haste and instantaneous, fleeting grounding in which we live. The spiritual awareness and growth that mark spiritual formation take place in processes that may very well not even be chronologically measureable. They take place in what is referred to as kairotic time, known from the Greek of the New Testament as "the right time, in the fullness of time." Spiritual formations take place within us dementia caregivers as our very here and now experiences tease the edge of eternity.

Meditation Nineteen

Unbidden

JUST AS OUR CIRCUMSTANCE as caregiver with our Beloved on this journey has not been a matter of personal choice—this came upon us, and we said Yes!—so too are those moments of graceful gift, wherein some solace appears in the midst of our weariness. This is the strange quality of the unbidden: as we focus our attention, appropriately so, on the immediacy of meeting the needs at hand, unmediated realities drop in on us. We're not asking for these graces, or even seeking them, yet they occur.

There are numbers of those we refer to as mystics who report similar experiences. As noted earlier, Hildegard von Bingen is one of the more familiar, and popular, visionaries within the canons of those who have been gifted with insight or wisdom in the midst of pain, anxiety, suffering. As might be expected in assessing the life and personality of such a complex and impressive medieval woman, whose notoriety was broadcast in her own time, there has been an ongoing critique of her recounted experience. No less than Oliver Sacks, well known neurologist and voluminous writer, attributed her visions to coping with migraine attacks.[1] Others, like Matthew Fox, former Roman Catholic and now Episcopal priest, theologian, activist and writer, who are more patient with

1. Hozeski, *Hildegard*, "Foreword."

85

such personal faith- and witness-driven account narratives, accept her statements at face value.[2] Without engaging in judging the particular quality of her visions—hey, they could have been both, right?—let's simply note again how she ordinarily describes her graceful visions occurring:

> In the year 1141 . . . when I was forty-two years and seven months old, a burning light coming from heaven poured into my mind. Like a flame which does not burn but rather enkindles, it inflamed my heart and my breast, just as the sun warms something with its rays. And I was able to understand books suddenly, the psaltery clearly, the evangelists and the volumes of the Old and New Testament, but I did not have the interpretation of the words of their texts nor the division of their syllables nor the knowledge of their grammar. . . . I truly saw those visions; I did not perceive them in dreams, nor while sleeping, nor in a frenzy, nor with the human eyes or with the external ears of a person, nor in remote places; but I received those visions according to the will of God while I was awake and alert with a clear mind, with the innermost eyes and ears of a person, and in open places. There may be a reason why I received those visions in this manner, but it is difficult for a human person to understand why.[3]

Difficult to understand, indeed. And yet the experience of unbidden insight seems fairly common among reflective spiritual mentors. For example, the entirety of *Interior Castle*, Teresa of Avila's now classic reflection of the prayerful soul—or perhaps, soulful prayer!—seems to be an expansion of a thought that simply occurred to her as she fretted over the assignment given her by her superiors to write such a treatise. The dynamic associated with such immediate insight is quite unlike that associated with the result of careful or scholarly or research-oriented preparation for some clearly understood task. It is, rather, the dynamic that has caught our attention as caregivers: an unconstrained thrust of light into our darkness from an unknown source. It is not rational, yet

2. Hozeski, *Hildegard*, "Foreword."
3. Hozeski, *Hildegard*, ch. 9.

neither is it irrational. It seems illogical yet has pursued a logical course on the way to our consciousness.

As Hildegard has noted of her peculiar gift, she "hears the light."[4] Impossible? Or simply the impossible possibility?

Listen.

Late in our journey, my Beloved, after a few hours' outing together, quite lost in herself and wearied by the venture, turned to me while I was driving us back to Namaste Alzheimer's Center after what would then become our last jaunt off campus from her care facility.[5] With great precision, she said, "Everything is too large today. Everything is too large." Unbidden, an insight into how Ann was experiencing our shared time; a gift in grasping how the ordinary world was unfolding in her diminishing, yet extraordinary mind.

Listen.

One of our sons, Peter, had joined me one afternoon for a visit with his mother at Namaste. He was in his late twenties. One of the other residents in Ann's unit happened to have been one of Peter's pediatricians two decades previous. The good doctor, as Oliver Sacks says in one of his patient write ups, now had "fallen upon such evil days,"[6] and had not spoken a word for many, many months. He had developed gibberish aphasia and roamed the common room softly muttering unintelligible monosyllabic sounds. When Peter entered the room, the noncommunicative physician approached him, took him by the hand, and led him to the brightest window area available, gently rolled up Peter's sleeves, still mumbling incoherently. He actually examined him, then looked up and said, loudly and clearly, "Peter, your eczema is greatly improved!" He then dropped Peter's arms and returned to his ramble and aphasia. I will make no comment here, as we did not then, when we were gifted witnesses to a thundering miracle of clarity in the midst of chaos.

Unbidden.

Simple acceptance is available to us. Perhaps we will be gifted in accepting.

4. Hozeski, *Hildegard*, ch. 33.
5. This experience is related in greater detail in Ewing, *Tears*, 75–76.
6. Sacks, "Dementia Patient."

Meditation Twenty

Humility

PERHAPS THERE IS SOME nuanced difference between humility and being humbled. If so, it is lost to us dementia caregivers. Being humbled is our version of humility. However, humility is one of the spiritual "virtues" much addressed by contemplative writers; humility is proffered as one of the spiritual states to attain for those who seek any form of enhanced spirituality.

However, Bernard of Clairvaux, in his *Commentary on the Song of Songs*, does comment on both humility and being humbled, suggesting they are spiritually intertwined:

> It is only when humility warrants it, that great graces can be obtained; hence, the one to [receive these graces] is first humbled by correction, that by humility [one] may merit them. And so when you perceive that you are being humiliated, look on it as the sign of a sure guarantee that grace is on the way. . . . There are some who meet humiliation with rancor, some with patience, some again with cheerfulness. The first are culpable, the second are innocent, the last just. Innocence is indeed a part of justice, but only the humble possess it perfectly.[1]

1. Bernard, *Commentary*, Sermon 34, 226.

Bernard is speaking to monks in their state of vowed obedience, yet there is some reverberation in his words that is like the sound of dementia caregiving.

Francis de Sales, who deliberately advocates spiritual formation for those not in cloistered life, when promoting humility distinguishes true humility from false in his *Introduction to the Devout Life*:

> We often make-believe to run away and hide ourselves, merely to be followed and sought out; we pretend to take the lowest place, with the full intention of being honorably called to come up higher. But true humility does not affect to be humble, and is not given to make a display in lowly words. It seeks not only to conceal other virtues, but above all it seeks and desires to conceal itself. . . . Never cast down your eyes without humbling your heart; and do not pretend to wish to be last and least, unless you really and sincerely mean it.[2]

Some of us dementia caregivers, no doubt, would very much like to "run away and hide ourselves," but there is no "make-believe" space to do that. Nor would we, in our circumstances, be touting a false humility, "merely to be followed and sought out." Listen, though, to the dynamics here; they are pertinent to realizing a spiritual gift in the ordinary behaviors of caregiving.

The "hiding" Francis speaks to in this context is the manner in which a bloated or ego-driven spiritual leader were to withdraw from immediate social view, while harboring a desire to be found, and praised for their—in this case—false humility. The entire scenario is a fanciful luxury for us caregivers. There is no time to plot anything other than the next engaging presence being asked of us. The only "pretending" we ever do is more than likely to be in those moments of creative diversion we invent in order to draw down the Beloved's anxiety. Our "pretending" is entirely contextual and devoted to the Beloved. And we certainly entertain no vision of being exalted. The pace is too swift, in the topsy-turvy world of

2. de Sales, *Introduction*, pt. 3, ch. 5.

slowly evolving dementia, to imagine that our journey with the Beloved is directed to a "higher" place.

And yet what Francis attempts to describe as "true humility" is exactly where we find ourselves. However, the striking difference in context is that we have not striven to be here. We are brought to our knees, metaphorically and some days actually, within the simple unfolding of our daily hours of attendance and presence to the Beloved. We did not commit ourselves to this journey with any sense of achievement outside of this attendance and presence. We gave ourselves to this compassionate care. We are not "affecting to be humble." We are humbled . . .

We are humbled by the sheer impossibility of our meeting the vast needs at hand. We are humbled by the weariness we feel in body, mind, spirit, when the demanding day and night is not yet half tick-tocked away, with no end in sight. We are humbled by our inability to see beyond the immediacy of the moment, yet knowing the moment shall turn. And yet we do . . .

We meet the needs at hand. We breathe and behave beyond our weariness. We blink moist eyes and face the next moment as we have faced the last. What we do and manage and enact as caregivers is impossible. And we do it. Again mindful of Joseph Sittler's "impossible possibility," our very behaviors lift up concretely what Francis only theorizes as "true humility." Not having chosen to be caregiver to our Beloved, we are caregiver to our Beloved.

Being placed—not so much against our will, as against our imagining and dreams—beside the Beloved on this inconceivable dementia journey was perhaps the entry into humility, into being humbled. Humbled by circumstance and simple reality. Having come from beyond us, we first had options of denial or aversion or hiding before us. But not for long . . .

Saying Yes! engaged us quickly in the wisdoms and practices of caregiving. In the imminence of what lay ahead of us, we most likely were not even close to articulating the spiritual reality into which we were entering. Choosing to meet the impossible and to dedicate ourselves to the course of dementia caregiving was to accept a gift. We may not have seen it that way, yet now that is our choice: to realize that we were given, from beyond ourselves and our life-planning, the opportunity to be humbled in person, in physical strength, in spiritual desire, and in the ability to know we had so taken for granted. Or as the phrase is often punned upon, "taken for granite"—the rock beneath our feet became sand in a veritable instant. Our reality changed, and we had not asked for this graceful gift. That we might reframe painful, scorching loss as gift is one of those spiritual matters that come not only, but perhaps especially, to caregivers. There are other human experiences in which that transformative shift might occur—a fatal diagnosis of any kind, a horrid and tragic accident or military event, unforeseen financial disaster—yet within our dementia journey with the Beloved, the humbling of very self in the care now given is a spiritual gift unbidden, realized, if you will, in the next breath you draw . . .

Meditation Twenty-One

Intimacy

URGINGS TOWARDS SPIRITUAL FORMATION are often put in terms of increasing intimacy between the seeker and the Beloved. Contemplative and mystic writers are wont to liken their spiritual journey to an interior path leading to a more and more profound relationship with the Beloved. Through friendship, to affection, to love, to surrender, to union with the sacred, the passage these writers have chosen is described as a trajectory of ever deepening communion. From the thin vapors of an inquisitive faith, they move into thicker, denser environments of intimacy with the object of their holy desire.

The various way stations at which they pause along their journey are familiar to dementia caregivers. As we develop capacities to be our Beloved's compass, clock, and consciousness, the loss within the Beloved slowly becomes our soulful gain. Where once the dynamics of the Beloved's person and values and behaviors were displayed, there stand we, now doubly formed in graces of an inward intimacy. Our partnership with the Beloved is slowly transformed into an interior accord with the Beloved. What had been physical intimacy with the Beloved is now experienced as a soulful union.

The entirety of Teresa of Avila's *Interior Castle* can be read as an inward path to an ultimate intimacy with the castle keep, the Lord of the castle, and of her soul. From her befuddled beginnings in her assigned task—"I do not feel that the Lord has given me either the spirituality or the desire for it"[1]—she moves her Carmelite sisters in faith through six *moradas* ("rooms," though translated also as "mansions") into the seventh, where union with the Holy is consummated.

Teresa writes there, that the Lord "told her it was time she took upon her His affairs as if they were her own."[2] She enfolds, as we dementia caregivers do likewise, the Beloved into her soulful self. Plying "Spiritual Betrothal" and "Spiritual Marriage" as her model, Teresa speaks of this dynamic as resulting in "two who are united so that they cannot be separated anymore."[3] She refers to death . . . as do we.

Contemplative writers who choose to go there, do not shy away from sensual and sexual imagery as the explicit framing for the implicit union of the soulful seeker and the Beloved. Perhaps the most vivid poet among these mystics is Mechthild of Magdeburg. Among her soaring adorations of her Beloved, we find this paeon:

> Lord, you are my lover,
> My desire,
> My flowing fount,
> My sun,
> And I am your reflection.[4]

Among her prayers, this:

> Ah Lord, love me passionately, love me often, and love me long. For the more passionately you love me, the purer I shall become. The more often you love me, the more beautifully I shall become. The longer you love me, the holier I shall become here on earth.[5]

1. Teresa of Avila, *Interior Castle*, 212.
2. Teresa of Avila, *Interior Castle*, 213.
3. Teresa of Avila, *Interior Castle*, 213.
4. Mechthild, *Flowing Light*, bk. 1, sec. 4.
5. Mechthild, *Flowing Light*, bk. 1, sec. 23.

Bernard of Clairvaux is also well known for his near-erotic language of spirituality. His *Commentary on the Song of Songs* is a carefully written expansion of the eighty-six-sermon series he preached in less complex and more straightforward form to his fellow monks in 1115 CE.[6] Just as does his Hebrew biblical source, the Song of Songs, he lifts up sensual language of passionate love as the mark of spiritual formation, the language of lovemaking as the mark of inward, spiritual intimacy with the Beloved. From "Sermon 2":

> Not one of the prophets makes an impact on me with his words. But he, the one whom they proclaim, let him speak to me, "let him kiss me with the kiss of his mouth." I have no desire that he should approach me in their person, or address me with their words . . . rather in his own person "let him kiss me with the kiss of his mouth;" let him whose presence is full of love, become "a spring inside me, welling up to eternal life." Shall I not receive a richer infusion of grace from him whom the Father has anointed . . . provided that he will bestow on me the kiss of his mouth? . . . An unreserved infusion of joys, a revealing of mysteries, a marvelous and indistinguishable mingling of the divine light with the enlightened mind, which, joined in truth to God, is one spirit with him. With good reason then I avoid trucking with visions and dreams; I want no part with parables and figures of speech; even the very beauty of the angels can only leave me wearied. For my Jesus utterly surpasses these in his majesty and splendor. Therefore I ask of him what I ask of neither man nor angel: that he kiss me with the kiss of his mouth.[7]

In "Sermon 8," Bernard suggests this intimacy is on the same level as the relationship of the three Persons of the Holy Trinity, and in "Sermon 9," he further expands on suckling the breasts of the Beloved:

---

6. McGuire, "St. Bernard's Preaching."

7. Bernard, *Commentary*, Sermon 2.

Everything in the world indeed will come to an end, an end from which there is no return. Not so, however, the breasts [of the bride] we have spoken of. For when these have been drained dry, they are replenished again from the maternal fount within, and offered to all who will drink . . . the numbers who drink of them, however great, cannot exhaust their content; their flow is never suspended, for they draw unceasingly from the inward fountains of love. The accumulating praises of the breasts come to a climax in the perfume of the ointments, because they not only feed us . . . but shed around them like a pleasing aroma the repute of good deeds.[8]

And in "Sermon 23 (continued)," addressing intimacy with the bridegroom king in his bedrooms, he exhorts hearers and readers "to know that no maiden, or concubine, or even queen, may gain access to the mystery of that bedroom which the Bridegroom reserves solely for her who is his dove, beautiful, perfect and unique."[9]

Bernard of course speaks "symbolically," even while feigning dislike for vision and metaphor. For him and his formation, spiritual intimacy has as its foundation the ordinary experience of physical and emotional intimacy. The latter, for dementia caregivers, can also provide a profound movement into that intimacy which has no better descriptor than "spiritual."

How else to speak of the union fashioned within our daily, hourly embrace of the Beloved's being and need, absorbed into our own presence. Quietly, unbidden, even as a stranger in our Beloved's faltering sight and association, we emerge from the fog of perception as a solid, intimate soulmate . . . at last.

Father Thomas Keating states this even more succinctly: "Whatever degree of divine union we may reach bears no proportion to our effort. It is the sheer gift of divine love."[10]

---

8. Bernard, *Commentary*, Sermon 2.

9. Bernard, *Commentary*, Sermon 23 (continued).

10. Keating, *Open Mind*, 132.

Meditation Twenty-Two

Love

LOVE HAS THREADED ITS way through most every one of these reflections on the pain and the gift of dementia caregiving. The dominance of love in contemplatives' spiritual counsel and advocacy is clear as well. The love so spoken and lauded is love known in both the Hebrew and Greek foundational sacred literature as forms of בהא (*ahav*), translated into, and written as, forms of ἀγάπή (*agapé*). Unlike our English word "love," the deliberateness of the Hebrew and Greek words do not point to a range of emotions, but to a singular behavioral commitment to actual loving.

It is often explained that agapé love is "unconditional love." That simplistic explanation, however, does not capture the way agapé love is actually conditioned. Agapé love, if you will, is tempered in the heat of circumstance that calls up loving out of deep identification with the Beloved, the object of love; it is "conditioned," in this case, by caregivers' radical squandering of their being and presence.[1] All, all, is given over to the Beloved. Perhaps "unconditional" might remain as a reference to this mode of loving, but the term falls short of acknowledging how caregivers exercise no intention to abandon conditional dynamics, those that ordinarily

---

1. "Radical squandering" is the delightfully insightful turn of phrase Cynthia Bourgeault uses while reflecting on "self-emptying love" in *Wisdom*, 64, 69–70 to describe the love made visible in Jesus of Nazareth's life and ministry.

circumscribe how humans dispense and express "love." Dementia caregivers appear to make no conscious decision to shape or re-shape their love and loving. We don't think about it. We love.

As Norman Wirzba has put it, commenting on the love that the assassinated Salvadorian bishop Óscar Romero walked into the life of the faithful in his charge, "love does not allow people to flee or shield themselves from the pain or the troubles of this life. Genuine lovers move deeply into the life-and-death dramas of this world, like a plant that sinks roots deep into fertile soil, and there give themselves wholly to the flourishing of life. To with-hold oneself from love is to withhold oneself from participating in a complete life. . . . Love is the outbound movement that trains people to . . . kindly embrace the world."[2]

Caregivers have been granted the gift of embracing the world of the Beloved. We have been graced, from beyond ourselves, to become a fountain, not only of holy tears, but as well, a bubbling spring of agapé love.

Our love is reciprocated in unexpected and odd ways. Odd, that is, in contrast to the more ordinary loving exchanges between lovers in the swirling human experiences that do not include inti-macy within dementia and dementia care. I am fairly certain that the experience I have had with my Beloved, while unique to me and Ann, is shared by many dementia caregivers. Often, towards the end of our journey, while Ann could still speak, she would turn to me during our visits at Namaste to say, to me, the safe stranger, "I love you . . ." Wherever she was in her outwardly diminishing world, her interior world held the heat and fire and light of expe-rienced love, and she fiercely spoke to and of and from that place. We have not loved for our own welfare, but for the welfare of the Beloved . . . and this love is mirrored back, for it is, indeed, "stron-ger than death."

Bernard of Clairvaux, who reflected long and devoutly on the mysterious love which bound the broken faithful into the beauty of being lovers, dove deeply into the waters of the love proclaimed in the Song of Songs, from which that piercing witness leaps: "Love

2. Rohr, "Daily Meditations," Feb. 21, 2023.

is stronger than death." He looks out onto the comrades within his order and muses:

> Let love enkindle your zeal, let knowledge inform it, let constancy strengthen it. Keep it fervent, discreet, courageous. See it is not tepid, or temerarious, or timid. . . . The love of the heart relates to a certain warmth of affection, the love of the soul to energy or judgment of reason, and the love of strength can refer to constancy and vigor of spirit, the full and deep affection of your heart, love with your mind wholly awake and discreet, love with all your strength, so much so that you would not even fear to die for love. . . . Let your love be strong and constant, neither yielding to fear nor cowering at hard work. Let us love affectionately, discreetly, intensely. We know that the love of the heart, which we have said is affectionate, is sweet indeed, but liable to be led astray if it lacks the love of the soul. And the love of the soul is wise, indeed, but fragile without that love which is called the love of strength.[3]

Bernard is not theorizing. He, like so many contemplatives, is caught in the throes of what he is experiencing, a raptured way of being in the world, an overwhelming, soulful exchange with the Beloved that simply descends as light into the darkness of the journey.

So too, Hildegard's visions, bedazzled with blinding light, render love as the vehicle of splendid goodness and care. She speaks of the "burning torch" of love, the love which is "the color of hyacinth," making all things bright around it. To what end? That we "may faithfully succor each and every needy person . . . clothed with the tunic of the sweetness of God . . . to shine forth with devotion, action, and experience to all people with righteous light." And in so being in the world as the presence of love, the lover "may reject death and come through to life."[4]

What mystics and contemplatives "see" and advocate for the unfolding of love in the world is actually the makeup of a dementia caregiver's extraordinary day. Our behavior says, "I love you,"

3. Bernard, *Commentary*, Sermon 20.
4. Hozeski, *Hildegard*, ch. 33.

and the Beloved returns from death to live, with us, here, now, in unbidden, graceful love.

Part Seven

Completions

PERHAPS IT HAS NOT been helpful, or accurate, to describe our caregiving journey as having "a beginning, a middle, and an end." Endings are odd moments. We help ourselves through death, for example, by holding the experience as a flowing passage, another beginning, or perhaps as an extended middle. How often "commencement" addresses, too, are cast as just that, beginnings as something very humanly developmental actually ends.

Nonetheless, there is this complex time marked decisively by the Beloved's death. The Beloved, long gone in many of the aspects of ordinary knowing and yet revealed in newer configurations of being as the stricken Beloved, is now memorialized in whatever ways we find to honor the deceased, quietly for some of us, publicly for some of us, given over to traditions and family practices for some of us. There is now a mark on the calendar, and in our hearts. There is a noted, remembered "time" which appears, electric and pulsing, in unbidden, scorching moments across all our time.

This peculiar kairotic time is now lodged in our life's journey, and we may return to it on our scheduled spiritual praxis or be returned to it by turns and events unforeseen. The passage is not captured with the word "ending," although there is within the Beloved's passage from our physical presence a completion: a completion of our daily caregiving, though its impact lingers, perhaps forever; a completion of the routines we had come into stride with beside our afflicted beloved; a completion of the Beloved's presence for and with and by us.

The completion within this time has oddly stitched fragments around the edges of our experience. Our journey continues, and we may again be lost for a time. And then again found.

Meditation Twenty-Three

Beyond Space and Time

THE SO-CALLED "SIGNS AND symptoms" of Alzheimer's disease actually become the realities within which we caregivers and our Beloveds live, daily. Whether we learn to live with these realities as modalities of spiritual formation or not, they are nonetheless the markers of the world we inhabit with our Beloved. Discomfiting, disorienting, confusing, unsettling, painful, and the source of our deepening sorrow—all this.

In our waking lives with the Beloved, we have entered a dimension beyond ordinary space and time; time is actually only here and now, space is wherever our Beloved claims it to be. We are pilgrims in the new land of forgetfulness.

And yet . . .

We have mused on how contemplatives and mystics regard the contours of our land of forgetfulness as the new ordinary of their lives in awareness and mindfulness, of their sought-out life in union with the Holy. I suspect few of us dementia caregivers think of ourselves as contemplatives or mystics. Nonetheless, we have, like them, sometimes reluctantly, sometimes willfully, entered a new way of being in the world. An invitation to entertain spiritual formation within this unexpectedly renewed life is always extended. What if we were to accept the invitation? Even for a quick drop in . . .

Contemplatives, after all, do not speak of life beyond space and time as a steady state universe. If anything, the gift of inhabiting this freed and unitive environment with the Holy is fleeting, unbidden, and still mysterious. As Father Thomas Keating has put it, experiences of interior transformation "are transient and are not the end of the journey"; some might awaken to a sense of the indwelling of the Holy "in great abundance," while others may "have to live most of the time without them."[1] In like manner, John of the Cross, commenting on a reference in the Song of Songs to "swift-winged birds," rues the way in which these moments of spiritual insight and satisfaction are subject to "wanderings of the imagination . . . for these digressions are quick and restless in flying from one place to another."[2]

Difficult and challenging as it may be, living in these moments and engagements with the Beloved beyond space and time carries with it the possibility of immersive presence. There is harm to be done in "correcting" the Beloved when she or he looks us in the eye and calls us by the name of the dead. There is harm to be done in "reorienting" the Beloved to her or his "real" place in the world when we are invited to join them in some long-ago picnic or party or moment of treasured recall, as if it were here, now.

Perhaps there is no harm at all, however, in abandoning our ordinary time and space to enter the world of our Beloveds in the land of forgetfulness, to be present with them in these moments beyond space and time. When we "return," perhaps we shall have been enlightened in the freedoms of this unfettered place.

Immersed in their visions, Hildegard of Bingen and Julian of Norwich were simply open and available to what was presented to them, odd and fiery and unworldly as the visions may have been. They did not flinch. Nor should we, when beckoned into the land of forgetfulness by our Beloveds. What the Beloved sees and describes may be just as bizarre and unconnected to where

1. Iachetta, *Daily Reader*, Feb. 23.
2. John of the Cross, *Works*, 553.

I happen to be at the moment as these "showings" were to these contemplative visionaries. That does not make the Beloved's world any the less real or lived. When Ann asked me to join her "in the sound of the flower," I did my utmost to do so. I cannot report on the "sound," yet I still relish the moment I was invited into the form and shape of her world, one which I could only enter through the gates of abandoned perceptions, forsaken constructions of "reality." There is a Presence in the behaviors of being present, and perhaps it is the Holy.

I have recounted in *Tears in God's Bottle* how our four-year-old granddaughter Lisa created a sacred space with her beloved granny when Ann was deep, deep into the land of forgetfulness, non-communicative and lost to us.[3] Lisa had done so during a visit at Namaste, when I had honored her request, "Grandpa, will you please go away now? I want my own private time with Granny." We were outside on a lovely sunny summer afternoon, strolling around a peaceful duck pond on the premises. I saw to it that Ann was seated safely on a bench by the pond, and retreated, watching this "private time" unfold. Lisa first pranced in front of her granny, showing off her hair bow, then softly took her granny's face into her little hands, making eye-to-eye contact while she prattled on, and then crawled onto her granny's lap. Ann glowed, smiled. There was light there, where there had only been darkness. The ground was made sacred by their interaction; the moment was holy.

When later in the day, on our drive to her home, I asked Lisa what she had been talking about, what she had been doing in her time with Granny, she seemed befuddled, even aghast at my question. "Grandpa," she said, with some puzzlement about my not understanding, "I wasn't talking about anything, I wasn't doing anything. I was just loving her."

How did I not get it? This child had entered totally into the land of forgetfulness and returned with the experience and blessing of the Holy—that beyond space and time, there is Love.

---

3. Ewing, *Tears*, ch. 16.

Meditation Twenty-Four

Letting Go

LOVING THE BELOVED IN the land of forgetfulness is a form of letting go; it is an anticipation of what will be the final letting go, at the end of the caregiving journey. Contemplatives interlace the profundities of love and death in sometimes exultant ways. "Spiritually speaking," John of the Cross writes, "the suffering of love is like dying." He equates contemplation itself with love and loving, and imagines the death of those who so love as "sweet and gentle." The "mystical ladder of divine love" and contemplation culminates in the completeness of love—that is, death.[1]

Julian of Norwich repeatedly offers her near-death suffering as a vehicle for sacred love. She confirms that a blessing of her having lived through her desired yet deeply painful illness is that she might love more completely into her death. The fullness of love, she claims, "transforms our sorrowful dying into holy, blessed life." And in another paean to love, Julian of Norwich contends that "when the soul has become nothing for love . . . then it is able to receive spiritual rest." So, without love we cannot live, yet the fullness of love is comprehended finally in death.[2]

---

1. John of the Cross, *Works*, 500, 440–45, 514, 653–54.
2. Julian of Norwich, *Showings*, 127, 132, 134, 263, 342–43.

In some similar sense, we dementia caregivers love into and unto death with our Beloved. We have already abandoned "self" for the Beloved; we have melded our waking desires into the Beloved's. While we are not contemplatives and mystics, these we have been citing would understand, perhaps even praise, the path we have taken into the land of forgetfulness. And just as, say, Julian of Norwich and John of the Cross take great pains to unwrap the various nuances and characters of love, so we too have experienced our loving. For example, our soulful movement from rote obligation to the Beloved, to selfless and compassionate loving beyond space and time, is not only generative and transformative. It is, beyond our ken and willfulness, a brush with the gentle presence of the Holy.

Over thirty years ago the late Sherwin Nuland wrote of dementia caregiving in a manner that is still poignantly focused on our caregiving experience:

> All along the way, family members have been experiencing feelings of ambivalence, helplessness, and crisis. They fear what they are seeing, as well as what they have yet to see. . . . And yet, it is always so hard to let go. . . . Alzheimer's is one of those cataclysms that seems designed specifically to test the human spirit. . . . The only rescue comes with the death of a person they love. . . . For the survivors, the concourse of existence has forever become less bright and less direct. . . . There is no dignity in this kind of death. . . . If there is wisdom to be found, it must be in the knowledge that human beings are capable of the kind of love and loyalty that transcends not only the physical debasement but even the spiritual weariness of the years of sorrow.[3]

If we might echo John of the Cross, spiritually speaking Dr. Nuland captured the soulful poignancy of love unto death, and through death. So too has, if I may so describe him, the contemplative surgeon Atul Gawande. In his quiet and sometimes disturbing meditations on death, dying, and medicine, he, like every one of

3. Nuland, *How We Die*, 105–6.

Part Seven: Completions

us caregivers, focuses on "what it's like to be creatures who age and die, how medicine has changed the experience, and how it hasn't, where our ideas about how to deal with our finitude have got the reality wrong."[4]

Gracious and caring as these good doctors are, and immersed as they have been in death and dying not only professionally, but as well in searing personal intimacy, they write to us and for us in the general. We have lived, or are living, or will live, with the specific realities of death and dying, in consummate relationship with our Beloved. Death has not been, nor will it be, conceptual, abstract; rather, it is relational. Perhaps this is where we caregivers actually have one up on the contemplatives and mystics we have visited: we have, or will have, completed the journey through the land of forgetfulness unto the death of the Beloved. Whether we "got the reality wrong" or not, whether we have been, or are, sorely wounded by the soulful experience of our caregiving, we are forever marked as a lover, for whom the letting go of the Beloved was more than arduous. It began with a diagnosis and misgivings, proceeded through the horrors of dying by sentences and inches of self, and has ended with a farewell that began months, sometimes years, before death.

Letting go has been the spiritual diet of the desert in which we have feasted with the Beloved. Perhaps this letting go, now, shall become our entrance into what has been only imagined and advocated by our contemplative sources, a sacred place newly mapped in our souls, and where we taste the sweetness of the Holy.

4. Gawande, *Being Mortal*, 9.

Epilogue:
And Could It Be?

Could it be? Could it be that personal, spiritual transformation is possible during our caregiving journey into and through the land of forgetfulness? Could it be that we are given the opportunity to hold the Beloved in our memories in a radically different way at the end of the journey? Could it be that how we saw the Beloved at the beginning of our caregiving experience was the result of our shock and fear only? That we emerge from the daily walk with the Beloved not only with a newly birthed view of the Beloved, but as well with a newly birthed self?

Some dementia caregivers have already answered a resounding Yes! to these "could it be?" musings.[1] Here, I am asking that we all might explore a path of renewal. It is a low risk undertaking. The higher risk we are already engaged in is caregiving itself, and we seem to be doing OK with that risk. We are surviving, where our Beloved has not. We have survived, when our Beloved has not, disappearing on us before we were ready.

I remember the prescience of my Beloved in something she said to me shortly before we sought medical counsel for insight into the oddness of her behavior, memory, and confusion. "I don't think," Ann mused, "I'm going to make it to the end of my life."[2]

---

1. For example, Hogan, "Gift of Dementia."
2. Ewing, *Tears*, prologue, xi.

She didn't. The medical counsel resulted in a diagnosis: early onset dementia, Alzheimer's type.

It is initially unimaginable that a stunning diagnosis might also become a welcoming trailhead for the caregiver to enter upon a journey toward spiritual health and wellbeing. In these meditations we have attempted to unravel some of the complexities of dementia caregiving in their specifics, while paralleling that experience with unraveling some contemplatives' insights into the purposefulness of life in general. But is there more than just the quirkiness of language involved?

Certainly we caregivers are in no space, place, or condition from within which we could even speculate on the spirituality of the Beloved. Pointless; meaningless. Yet we are from time to time exquisitely tuned into our own spiritual state. As has been noted, that may first be recognized as despair, hopelessness, exhaustion of body and spirit, weariness of soul. From that place, we are prone to perceive the Beloved as a kind of embodied black hole into which our history, our future, our legacy is disappearing; and as in the heart of every galaxy, from which no light escapes.

With increasing intimacy with the Beloved, however, no matter how frayed and tattered that may be, there are invitations for us to frame our experience differently. Even should the Beloved mistrust us, there is an ultimate trust inlaid upon the experience for us. Even should the Beloved strike out in what appears to be anger—most likely this is fear and confusion, rather than anger—we might realize we are the safest person in the Beloved's tightening personal orbit to receive her or his anger.

There are, as noted in these meditations, other moments, day and night, marked by other qualities. An unwavering love and accepted dependency. From the gathering fog, a lucid quest for compass, clock, and map to be provided by us, the caregivers. Out of nowhere—though there is a somewhere beyond our ken and grasp—a smile, a hand squeeze. Small matters? No. Huge, actually, within the land of forgetfulness.

For us caregivers, the Beloved can emerge from the darkness as an angel of light, a beacon for our own life and living. Should it last a minute, it will have been a minute. And defying how we usually think of time passing, in this strange land of forgetfulness, that minute may cross all ordinary barriers to become the extraordinary, lasting newness of our look into and beyond our life and living.

Psalm 88 asks if there is "saving help in the land of forgetfulness?" The psalmist doesn't really answer. The question remains open and piercing. The psalm ends on a note of experiencing painful shunning, terror, and dread. The concluding words are, "my companions are in darkness." Yet along the way, the psalmist has twice claimed to have "cried out." The piercing question about the land of forgetfulness is not a condemnation, but a tearful lament; not final despair, but long, ongoing sorrow.

It is possible, still, that our sorrow is addressed from beyond us, by myriad voices embedded deeply in our broken human experience, voices that speak to us soulfully, not of delivery or escape, but of immersion into our Beloved's land of forgetfulness—a place where, yes, the Holy might live before us, within us, beside us. The Beloved, after all, is the Beloved . . .

Bibliography

Aeschylus. *Agamemnon*. Translated by George Theodoridis. www.poetryintranslation.com/PITBR/Greek/Agamemnon.php/textLinkTarget-YwdhbWVtbm9u.

Alzheimer's Association. "10 Early Signs and Symptoms of Alzheimer's and Dementia." https://www.alz.org/alzheimers-dementia/10_signs.

Amazingsusan. "101 Activities You Can Enjoy with a Person Living with Alzheimers Dementia." *My Alzheimer's Story* (blog), May 29, 2015. https://myalzheimersstory.com/2015/05/29/101-activities-you-can-enjoy-with-a-person-living-with-alzheimers-dementia/

Band, Arnold J. *Nahman of Bratslav: The Tales*. Mahwah, NJ: Paulist, 1978.

Barks, Coleman. *The Essential Rumi*. New York: Harper Collins, 2004.

Bayley, John. *Elegy for Iris*. Boston: G. K. Hall, 1999.

Bernard of Clairvaux. *Commentary on the Song of Songs by Saint Bernard of Clairvaux*. Edited by Darrell Wright. https://archive.org/details/st.bernardonthesongofsongs/mode/2up.

Bishop, Jane, and Mother Columba Hart, trans. *Hildegard of Bingen: Scivias*. Mahwah, NJ: Paulist, 1990.

Bourgeault, Cynthia. *The Wisdom Jesus: Transforming Heart and Mind*. Boulder, CO: Shambhala, 2008.

Brussat, Frederic, and Mary Ann Brussat. *Spiritual Literacy: Reading the Sacred in Everyday Life*. New York: Scribner, 1996.

Clayton, Ingrid. "Beware of Spiritual Bypass." *Psychology Today*, Oct. 2, 2011. www.psychologytoday.com/us/blog/emotional-sobriety/201110/beware-spiritual-bypass.

Clift, Eleanor. "The Long Goodbye." *Newsweek*, Oct. 1, 1995. https://www.newsweek.com/long-goodbye-184022.

Coleman, Janet. "Augustine's De Trinitate; on Memory, Time, and the Presentness of the Past." In *Ancient and Medieval Memories*, 101–12. Cambridge: Cambridge University Press, 1992.

Bibliography

Colledge, Edmund, and Bernard McGinn. *Meister Eckhart: The Essential Sermons, Commentaries, Treatises, and Defense.* Mahwah, NJ: Paulist, 1981.

de Sales, Francis. *Introduction to a Devout Life.* www.catholicspiritualdirection. org/devoutlife.pdf.

DiBaggio, Thomas. *Losing My Mind.* New York: Simon & Schuster, 2003.

Ewing, Wayne. *Tears in God's Bottle: Reflections on Alzheimer's Caregiving.* Bloomington, IN: AuthorHouse, 2002.

Fleming, Ursula, ed. *Meister Eckhart: The Man from Whom God Nothing Hid.* Springfield, IL: Templegate, 1990.

Gawande, Atul. *Being Mortal: Medicine and What Matters in the End.* New York: Henry Holt, 2014.

Harvard Health Publishing. "Warning Signs of Alzheimer's Disease." Harvard Medical School, Aug. 23, 2018. https://www.health.harvard.edu/healthy-aging/warning-signs-of-alzheimers-disease.

Hathaway, Bill. "Eyes Offer a Window into the Mystery of Human Consciousness." *Yale News,* Dec. 7, 2022. https://news.yale.edu/2022/12/07/eyes-offer-window-mystery-human-consciousness.

Hogan, Mary. "The Gift of Alzheimer's Disease." www.alz.org/blog/alz/november-2018/the-gift-of-alzheimer-s.

Hopkins, Gerard Manley. "God's Grandeur." www.poetryfoundation.org/poems/44395/god-grandeur.

Hozeski, Bruce, trans. *Hildegard von Bingen's Mystical Visions: Translated from Hildegard's Scivias.* Sante Fe, NM: Bear, 1995.

Iachetta, S. Stephanie, ed. *The Daily Reader for Contemplative Living: Excerpts from the Works of Father Thomas Keating.* New York: Continuum, 2003.

John of the Cross. *The Collected Works of St. John of the Cross.* Translated by Kevin Kavanaugh and Otilio Rodriguez. Washington, DC: ICS, 2017.

Julian of Norwich. *Showings.* Edited by Edmund Colledge, and James Walsh. Mahwah, NJ: Paulist, 1978.

Keating, Thomas. *Invitation to Love: The Way of Christian Contemplation.* New York: Continuum, 1992.

———. *Open Mind, Open Heart.* New York: Continuum, 1996.

Kempe, Margery. *The Book of Margery Kempe.* https://archive.org/details/bookofmargerykeoookemp.

Kierkegaard, Søren. *The Concept of Dread.* Princeton, NJ: Princeton University Press, 1946.

———. *Fear and Trembling.* New York: Penguin Classics, 1985.

Kiger, Patrick J. "10 Warning Signs of Dementia You Shouldn't Ignore." AARP, Oct. 2, 2019. Last updated Mar. 6, 2024. https://www.aarp.org/caregiving/health/info-2019/dementia-warning-signs.html?intcmp=AE-CAR-CRC-LL.

Kiper, Dasha. *Travelers to Unimaginable Lands: Stories of Dementia, the Caregiver, and the Human Brain.* New York: Random House, 2013.

Bibliography

Kushner, William. *When Bad Things Happen to Good People*. New York: Schocken, 1981.

Levine, Stephen, and Ondrea Levine. *Embracing the Beloved: Relationship as a Path of Awakening*. New York: Anchor, 1996.

————. *Who Dies? An Investigation of Conscious Living and Conscious Dying*. New York: Anchor, 1989.

Lilly. "Understanding the Signs." https://morethannormalaging.lilly.com/understanding-the-signs#know-the-difference.

Living Better 50. "Startling Number of Alzheimer's Caregivers Die Before Loved Ones." www.livingbetter50.com/silent-killer-startling-number-of-alzheimer's-disease-caregivers-die-before-loved-ones.

Mayo Clinic. "Alzheimer's Disease." Last updated Feb. 12, 2024. https://www.mayoclinic.org/diseases-conditions/alzheimers-disease/symptoms-causes/syc-20350447.

McGuire, Brian Patrick. "St. Bernard's Preaching with the Milk of Love." *Church Life Journal: A Journal of the McGrath Institute for Church Life* (blog), Aug. 20, 2021. https://churchlifejournal.nd.edu/articles/bernard-of-clairvauxs-preaching-with-the-milk-of-love/.

Mechthild of Magdeburg. *The Flowing Light of the Godhead*. Internet Archive. 1998. https://archive.org/details/flowinglightofgooooomech.

National Institute on Aging. "What Are the Signs of Alzheimer's Disease?" https://www.nia.nih.gov/health/alzheimers-symptoms-and-diagnosis/what-are-signs-alzheimers-disease.

Nicolas of Cusa. *The Vision of God*. Translated by Emma Gurney Salter. New York: Cosimo, 2007.

Nuland, Sherwin B. *How We Die: Reflections on Life's Final Chapter*. New York: Knopf, 1993.

Phillips, Suzanne M., and Monique D. Boivin. "Medieval Holism: Hildegard of Bingen on Mental Disorder." *Philosophy, Psychiatry, and Psychology* 14:4 (Dec. 2007): 359–68. https://muse.jhu.edu/article/249256.

Raab, Diane. "What Is Spiritual Bypassing?" *Psychology Today*, Jan. 23, 2019. https://www.psychologytoday.com/us/blog/the-empowerment-diary/201901/what-is-spiritual-bypassing.

Radden, Jennifer H. "Sigewiza's Cure." *Philosophy, Psychiatry & Psychology* 14:4 (Dec. 2007): 373–76. 2007. https://muse.jhu.edu/pub/1/article/249258.

Rohr, Richard. "Daily Meditations." www.cac.org.

Sacks, Oliver. "How Much a Dementia Patient Needs to Know." *New Yorker*, Mar. 4, 2019.

Saling, Joseph. "Understanding Alzheimer's Disease–Symptoms." WebMD, May 12, 2023. https://www.webmd.com/alzheimers/understanding-alzheimers-disease-symptoms.

Taragin, Rueven. "Being Aware of Awareness." *Jewish Press*, Aug. 19, 2022. www.jewishpress.com/judaism/torah/being-aware-of-awareness.

Teresa of Avila. *Interior Castle*. Translated by E. Allison Peers. New York: Doubleday, 1989.

Bibliography

Teske, Roland. "Augustine's Philosophy of Memory." In *Cambridge Companion to Augustine*, 148–58. Cambridge: Cambridge University Press, 2001. https://doi.org/10.1017/CCOL0521650186.012.

Walsh, James, ed. *The Cloud of Unknowing*. Mahwah, NJ: Paulist, 1981.

Welwood, John. *Toward a Psychology of Awakening*. Boulder, CO: Shambhala, 2000.

Wirzba, Norman. *Way of Love: Recovering the Heart of Christianity*. New York: HarperOne, 2016.

www.ingramcontent.com/pod-product-compliance
Lightning Source LLC
Chambersburg PA
CBHW050215270326
41914CB00003BA/420